WM 220
AW

ASSISTIVE TECHNOLOGY IN DEMENTIA CARE

Developing the role of technology in the care and rehabilitation of people with dementia
– current trends and perspectives

Edited by John Woolham

D1339094

ASSISTIVE TECHNOLOGY IN DEMENTIA CARE

Developing the role of technology in the care
and rehabilitation of people with dementia
– current trends and perspectives

First published in 2006 by
Hawker Publications Ltd, Culvert House, Culvert Road,
London SW11 5DH

Tel: 020 7720 2108 Fax: 020 7498 3023

Email: info@hawkerpublications.com

Website: www.careinfo.org

© 2006 Hawker Publications

All rights reserved. No part of this publication may be reproduced
transmitted in any form or by any means, electronic or mechanical,
including photocopy, recording, or any information storage and retrieval
system without permission in writing from the publishers.

British Library Cataloguing in Publication Data

A Catalogue in Publication Data
ISBN 1 874790 83 3

Cover design by Andy Jackson

KINGSWAY HOSPITAL
01848
LIBRARY
19.09.07
DERBY

Table of contents

Foreword

Professor Mary Marshall

This is a very useful book. John Woolham has made an invaluable contribution to better dementia care by collecting and editing these papers as well as adding his own wise commentary.

The Journal of Dementia Care has had an illustrious role in promoting the proper use of technology for people with dementia through journal articles, the Astrid Guide and the annual conferences on technology and dementia. This role is now enhanced by this book which makes some hard-earned expertise available to a wide audience.

People with dementia need to have access to technology as part of any care package, to the same extent as other groups who need help to remain independent. They need it to be provided in a thoughtful, sensitive and ethical way. This welcome book makes this more likely to happen.

1. Introduction

John Woolham

The idea to put together this book began at a Technology and Dementia Care conference organised by Hawker Publications in autumn 2003. The conference brought together a series of speakers whose work reflected a range of different perspectives on the theme of using technology in dementia care settings. The speakers all kindly agreed to develop their presentations so they could be published.

In addition to these conference speakers, whose work forms the largest part of this book, contributions were invited from others on important issues that were not covered at the conference.

The level of interest in the potential use of assistive technologies has grown since Technology Ethics and Dementia (Bjørneby et al 1999) and the ASTRID handbook (Marshall (ed.) 2000) offered the first practical guidance for practitioners and others on how best to use technology to support people with dementia and those who care for them. The dementia care 'community' within the U.K. has helped to pioneer the use of assistive technology, and a number of locally based projects have been set up throughout the UK (Curry et al 2001). Their number continues to grow.

There is now considerable awareness of the potential of assistive technologies to manage risks arising from the impairments caused by ageing and dementia. Some, particularly clinicians and those working in allied health care fields, are beginning to explore the use of technology in helping to manage chronic illness and long term conditions – including dementia – by preventing known risks but also by using technology to support monitoring and assessment activity to predict 'risky' behaviour or events. At the leading edge, academics have also begun to consider how new technologies might enable people with dementia to spend their leisure time in ways they find both pleasurable and meaningful. (Enable Project 2002, Independent Project 2005).

In tandem, there has been a rapid expansion in the number of products available from manufacturers and suppliers. At the same time these manufacturers have become aware that these new technologies need to reach new markets – social and health care commissioners and providers as well as the traditional local authority housing and housing associations to whom community alarm systems have been sold for many years.

Interest has not just been confined to academics, local professionals, and managers keen to improve the quality of life of people with dementia and their carers. Within England, influential reports by the Audit Commission (2001, 2004) and I&DeA (2003) have raised the profile of this area of work to a point where, at the time of writing, the Government's Green Paper on the future direction of social care - Quality Choice and Independence (Department of Health 2005a) emphasises a key role for technology in providing support to all users of social care services, not just those who are living with dementia. Further guidance on telecare was published by the Department of Health in July 2005. Similar guidance has also been published for Scotland and Wales.

The fact that assistive technology and telecare has gone from being a fringe interest of a few enthusiasts to mainstream thinking in little over five years is as astonishing as it is welcome.

However, the very success of this sector now means that there is a risk that the momentum will be 'technologically driven' in that the focus may be upon the acquisition and use of assistive technology as a panacea – without proper consideration of the needs, preferences and lifestyle of some end users. Two of the three main purposes of the Preventive Technology Grant (an £80 million funding stream for telecare provided for English local authorities from 2006) are stated to be to 'provide initial investment' and to 'co-ordinate demand to ensure industry grows as fast as possible' (Department of Health 2005b, p5). Performance indicators for telecare can reasonably be expected to follow for English local authorities. Person-centred approaches to the use of technology, consideration of ethical and legal issues and best practice may receive less attention and support amongst hard pressed managers who may wish to encourage the rapid mainstream use of technology across all service user groups; using it primarily to make budget savings and meet performance indicator targets.

In addition, the general direction of key legislation and guidance in England over the last few years is toward consumer-led approaches to service delivery which among other things enable service users to have a much greater degree of choice and control over their care than was the case a decade ago. Greater choice is likely to be a welcome step for many or most service users. However, the exercise of choice is also dependent on the capacity of those concerned. Where informed consent to the use of

technology is only possible with considerable support, or where it is not possible, it is important that the use of assistive technology should take place within a therapeutic context and there must be clear and robust ethical protocols before it is used. Without these, there remain real dangers that technology might be used as a substitute for social care, or to control behaviour for the benefit of someone other than the person with dementia rather than to genuinely support their independence. It would be very unsatisfactory outcome if, having pioneered the use of assistive and telecare technology within the UK, its use within the dementia care community were to become marginalised as a result of the mainstreaming process.

One way in which these potential risks can be addressed is by addressing some of the significant gaps in our understanding of what actually is 'best practice' in the use of technology in dementia care. For example:

- What kinds of organisational obstacles might be found, and how can they be overcome, by anyone setting up a local project or service? Will the Preventive Technology Grant available to local authorities after 2006 lead to the creation of a plethora of new local technology projects all of which will make similar mistakes, or will they learn from those who have hard won experience of confronting and tackling these issues?
- What's the legal framework that underpins the use of technology? Are we in danger of fulfilling George Orwell's predictions, or can the law be used to support and guide its use - and prevent its abuse?

- Can more be said about the ethical issues that must be understood by those working in this field or has it all been said?
- Does technology have to mean 'high tech' – and perhaps more expensive, more difficult to install and maintain and harder to use - or can low level technologies also play an important role in supporting someone who is living with dementia?
- What kinds of approaches to assessment will be needed to ensure that technology is used appropriately? How can practitioners develop their knowledge and skills to assess for assistive technology and avoid 'recipe' based approaches to assessment.

The contributions within this book are intended both to provoke thought and act as a source of reference for these issues. The contributors - academics, professionals and managers from a range of different occupational backgrounds - are all linked by a keen interest in dementia care issues and technology as well as a commitment to improving services for people with dementia and their carers.

The second chapter, by Marilyn Cash, challenges our idea of what assistive technology can mean. Her paper examines the potential of 'low level' assistive technologies. She considers what kinds of devices are available, explores the perceptions people with dementia, their carers and professionals have of technology, and reports on the impact that a selection of these technologies have had on the lives of people with dementia and their carers. Her paper concludes with a series of evidence based recommendations about the value of

these devices and the role of professionals in ensuring their best use.

The third chapter, by Christine Calder, reports on a project in South Lanarkshire designed to consider the value of technology in supporting the continuing independence of people with dementia. Her paper demonstrates clear benefits to the project's participants and ends with a series of statements offering practical advice to people interested in developing similar kinds of projects or services.

Whilst Calder's contribution reports on a project, chapters four and five, by Dyllis Faife and Eileen Askham respectively, reflect on the development of technology *services* – one in a local authority context and the other in a Housing Association. Both offer a clear analysis of obstacles, risks and achievements. Faife draws a useful distinction between the skills needed to establish a new project or service and those needed to develop this within mainstream settings. Her personal and very readable account of the challenges of establishing the Norfolk S.T.I.L. project will be of particular interest to service developers and managers. Askham's parallel account of the development of assistive technology and telecare services at Fold Housing Association in Northern Ireland demonstrate the commitment needed by pioneers when it may be easier to find reasons not to do something than to do them. Both contributions offer very useful practical guidance.

If the first four contributions offer essentially practical guidance, the remaining three chapters offer guidance of a different kind.

Chapter six, by Clive Baldwin, offers a fresh and deeper examination of ethics and the relationship between values and assistive technology in dementia care. He invites the reader to re-examine conventional wisdoms about the essential neutrality of technology. This makes both slightly unsettling but very rewarding reading. The paper suggests that conventional ethical frameworks are a particular frame of reference amongst others and explores the value of other frameworks in developing ethical approaches to the use of technology. One of the paper's conclusions is a plea for a more for 'proactive' approach to ethics, so that rather than responding to technological progress, greater consideration be made of the kinds of values that technology should reflect.

Chapter 7, by Michael Mandelstam, offers an overview of the law relating to the provision of assistive technology. The contribution is both timely and necessary as at the present time there are few published contributions in this area. The chapter is clearly written and provides very helpful summary of what is a considerable range of relevant law. Examples are used to illustrate the impact of law on practice and policy. Mandelstam argues that existing law is not, as might be supposed, a barrier to the creative use of technology to meet the needs of people with dementia, but demands a 'balanced' approach that is likely to support good practice.

The final chapter, by Stephen Wey, is not about technology *per se* but offers a theoretical basis for assessment and practice activity in the field of dementia care within which assistive technology is one component of a wider framework. The paper, which focuses on the subject of rehabilitation, is a reminder of the sensitivity, knowledge and skills needed by professionals – regardless of discipline - to understand the needs of someone

living with dementia. The chapter offers a standard for others to aim in relation to the use of assistive technology in dementia care. It's also a great antidote to practitioners suffering from over-exposure to performance indicators and other managerial tools.

Taken together, the contributions offered here should be useful to anyone committed to trying to use technology to sustain and improve the quality of life and level of independence of people living with dementia. They may also offer a useful introduction for those heading this way.

References

The Audit Commission., (2004) <u>Assistive Technology, Independence and Well-being</u> Audit Commission.

Bjørneby, S., Holthe, T., & Topo, P., (1999) <u>Technology, Ethics and Dementia.</u> Norwegian Centre for Dementia Research.

Curry, R., Wardle, D., & Tinoco, M.T., (2002) *The Use of Assistive technology to Support Independent Living for Older and Disabled People.* ICES/DH.

Department of Health, (2005a) <u>Independence Well-being and Choice.</u> Green Paper, Department of Health.

Department of Health, (2005b) Building Telecare in England.

European Union., Quality of Life and Management of Living Resources R&D programme: (2004) *The Enable Project.*

Engineering & Physical Sciences Research Council (2005) *The Independent Project: Investigating*

Enabling Domestic Environments for People with Dementia.

Improvement & Development Agency., (2003) Local E-Government Now. I&DeA & Socitim.

Marshall, M., (ed.) (2000) ASTRID: A Social and Technological Response to Meeting the Needs of People with Dementia and their Carers. Hawker, London.

2. Exploring the potential of existing low-key technological devices to support people with dementia to live at home

Marilyn Cash

Introduction

At Home with AT (Assistive Technology) was a two year research project which ended in December 2004. The research was funded by the Sir Halley Stewart Trust and was undertaken by Dementia Voice, Bristol, in partnership with Borough of Poole Social Services, Dorset County Council Social Care and Health Services, Bournemouth Borough Council Social Services and Dorset HealthCare NHS Trust. This chapter will provide the background to the research, give a brief outline of the research methodology, and discuss the findings from the research.

Aim of the research

The overall objective of At Home with AT (Assistive Technology) was to explore the potential of existing low-key technological devices, which are readily available, to support people with dementia and their carers in their own homes.

Background to the research

Promoting independence in old age and enabling older people to remain in their own homes are key aims of current government policy (Department of Health 2000 & 2001a). The role of 'electronic assistive technology' to support vulnerable people, such as those with dementia, has been acknowledged by The Integrated Community Equipment Services Initiative (Department of Health 2001b).

In the UK and Europe there are a growing number of initiatives and research focused on the needs of people with dementia using 'smart home' technology (Fisk 2001). However little work seems to have been done to explore the potential of 'low-level' assistive technological devices - those readily available for purchase - to support people with dementia and their carers in their own homes.

Defining assistive technology

Technology used in the homes of people with dementia is generally referred to as assistive technology for its ability to *'assist the person with dementia to live as normal a life as possible'*.

Marshall (2001: p. 130).

A number of definitions of assistive technology have been developed. Early definitions were based on the medical model of disability and focused on functional disability. Later definitions have moved away from the negative connotations of disability placing the emphasis on preserving and maintaining independence (Tinker 2003). Marshall defines assistive technology as

'any item, piece of equipment, product or system whether acquired commercially, off the shelf, modified or customised, that is used to increase, maintain or improve functional capabilities of individuals with cognitive, physical or communication disabilities'.

Marshall (ed.) (2000: p. 9).

A wide range of applications of assistive technology for people with dementia fall within this definition, including smart housing, telecare and low-level technology.

Low-level technology

For the purpose of this project 'low-level' technology is defined as any item, piece of equipment, product or system that is available on the open market that may have the potential to support people with dementia and their carers by enabling them to continue to live in their own homes.

Low-level assistive technological devices are at what Marshall (1999) describes as the 'DIY store' end of the market. These are available for purchase through high street stores, mail order catalogues and the internet and include:

- movement detectors
- carbon monoxide sensors
- light and motion sensitive night lighting
- anti - flood devices such as a bath or sink plug which opens as water pressure reaches pre-set levels.

The anticipated benefits of low level technological devices are that they:

- are readily available for purchase
- can be used in the existing home of the person with dementia
- do not require the installation of sophisticated computer equipment
- do not need to be linked in with call centre telephony and infrastructure
- can be easily removed or adapted as the needs of the person with dementia change.

Research methodology

The study used description and analysis of the perspectives of the key 'players' - people with dementia and their carers, professional care staff, local contractors and suppliers. Methods included semi-structured interviews with people with dementia and their carers, Home Improvement Agency (HIA) and DIY store staff, a self-completion questionnaire for social care and health professionals who referred people to the study and focus groups with carers and people with dementia as well as a range of health and social care professionals. Quantitative data was analysed using SPSS. Analysis included descriptive statistics, such as frequencies and cross tabulations. Qualitative data was thematically analysed. Local Research Ethic Committee (LREC) approval was obtained before the study began. The data was collected over a two year period and in two phases.

Phase I had two distinct aims. The first was to identify devices in the marketplace that might provide support to people with dementia and their carers. The second was to explore what people understand the terms 'assistive technology' or 'assistive device' to mean. In phase I of the study, focus groups and semi-structured interviews were used to gather data.

In phase 2 the aim was to monitor the impact of a selection of assistive devices chosen from the devices identified in phase I of the project in a sample of homes by evaluating the support provided by the devices to people with dementia and their carers.

Recruitment and time schedule for the trial of the device

A number of sources were used to recruit participants including memory clinics, social services, community mental health teams, primary mental health teams, voluntary agencies, sheltered housing providers and day centres.

Contact with participants followed a three stage process:

- obtaining consent and selecting a device to use

- visits or telephone calls to participants 1 week + post commencement of the trial
- home visits and interviews with the person with dementia and carer (N.B. not all carers participated in the interview process) 1 month + post commencement of the trial.

Participants who trialled the device for over a month were regarded as having completed the trial.

Participants

The criteria used to select people to take part in the study were that the person should have a dementia or have significant cognitive impairment or memory difficulties but have the ability to give continuing consent to take part in the study. In addition, those selected had to be receiving dementia services, have no recent history of psychiatric morbidity and not be involved in other research or drug trials. Finally, those selected had to have a carer who was in regular contact.

Details of potential participants who met these criteria were passed to the project with their permission

The consent process

The issue of obtaining informed consent from prospective research participants is an important consideration in research. In dementia care, informed consent is complicated by the cognitive problems and diminished autonomy and capacity or competence of people with dementia (Bjørneby & van Berlo 1997, Bjørneby *et al* 1999). However, lack of competence cannot be assumed just because a person has a diagnosis of dementia (Bartlett & Martin 2002, p. 51). Better skills in communication with people with dementia are pushing

back previously assumed limits (Marshall 2000 p. 42).

The consent procedure used in this project was based on the consent procedure described by Allan (2001). The information and consent process included a potentially lengthy orientation period during which time the researcher took time to establish a rapport with the person and to ensure that they understood the research aims and process described in the project information leaflet. This process was tailored to the individual needs of each person.

Phase 1.

Identification of assistive devices

A range of devices available for purchase on the open market were identified by the researcher from a wide variety of sources, including DIY stores, mail order catalogues and internet websites. A number of devices were selected from within this range for trial in the homes of people with dementia.

Device Functions	Types of Devices	Usage	Support
Safety	Lighting	Night-time lighting A simple plug in light with PIR which comes on at dusk and goes off at dawn or can be set so that it is operated by movement	To reduce falls at night, assist orientation, reduce anxiety.
Safety	Flood Prevention	'Magi Plug' Bath plug that prevents flooding by letting excess water out of the bath	To reduce worries, provide carer support
Door Alarm	Warning	A wire free door alarm Contacts fitted on a door send a signal to an alarm unit when the door is opened. This Indicates to a carer when a person has left a room, or gone outside the building	To provide carer support and reduce worries.
Reminder	Memo Minder	Message recorder and player. This device is operated by battery/AC adaptor and used to provide simple reminders. A chosen message is triggered automatically by movement.	To facilitate time orientation, support memory and reduce worries.
Reminder	Locator Device	A battery operated device that helps to find commonly misplaced items, e.g. keys. A key tag bleeps when the corresponding button on the locator device is pressed	To reduce worries and time spent looking for lost objects.
Reminder	Medication reminder	A battery driven medicine reminder that alarms at pre-set times. It reminds the person to take the drugs and provides the correct drugs in correct doses.	To reduce worries of forgetting to take medication.
Reminder	Telephone with pre-programmable buttons	Allows user to make a call by pressing a button next to the name of the person they wish to speak to.	To reduce anxiety and prevent social isolation.

Table 1. Devices chosen for At Home with AT.

Results

Focus group schedule and semi-structured interviews

The same topics were explored in both the focus groups and the semi-structured interviews.

- The definition of assistive technology proposed by Marshall was used to generate discussion around the topic.
- Two vignettes (short stories about hypothetical characters in specified circumstances) were used to prompt discussion.

Participants were asked to respond to the situation described in the vignette by stating what they would do, or how they imagine a third person would react to the circumstances portrayed. This approach was chosen because evidence suggests that commenting on a story is less personal than talking about direct experience. Vignettes are therefore useful in exploring potentially sensitive topics that participants might otherwise find difficult to discuss. The two vignettes used in this study are presented below.

Understanding of the terms 'assistive technology' and 'assistive devices'

Those taking part in focus groups or semi-structured interviews were generally unfamiliar with the terms 'assistive technology' and 'assistive devices' *"personally myself I haven't got a clue I don't know what it means at all"* (carer)

The term 'technology' was interpreted to mean something that was likely to be *"high tech" "electronic"* (carers) involving the use of *"computer type things"* (person with dementia).

A minority of carers indicated that "assistive devices" were devices that were used as *as aids to daily living* (carer) "*...to sort of help people that have got different troubles*" (carer)

Some carers and people with dementia indicated that they perceived assistive technology as something that would be used in an institutional setting, "*used in a big hospital*" (carer) by a professional, such as *"Doctors"* (person with dementia) or "*various technicians*" (person with dementia) rather than by an individual "*in their own home*" (ex-carer).

Health and social care professionals were more familiar with the terms 'assistive technology' and 'assistive devices', identifying them as aids that would provide support.

Sourcing assistive devices
Carers, people with dementia and health and social care professionals identified a range of potential sources where they thought they might be able to purchase assistive devices, including statutory services, electrical stores, DIY stores, mobility shops, mail order catalogues, and the voluntary sector. However they indicated that there is no consistent source of information available to them.

Some carers indicated that they would seek advice on devices from health and care professionals: "*I would start with my social worker because she seems to be a mine of information*". Others were uncertain about health and social care professionals' ability to provide information about accessing devices; "*professionals should be on the ball with that but whether they are or not I am not sure*".

Many social care professionals thought that whether or not they were able to

successfully locate a device to solve a particular problem depended on luck or being able to locate a colleague who had solved a similar problem. They indicated that there is no "*consistent source*" of information available to them and said that locating devices was "*hit and miss*".

These findings suggest that there is a need for greater promotion of the use of assistive technology and assistive devices amongst carers and people with dementia. The need for a managed national database of available assistive devices that is readily available to both health and social care professionals and carers is also indicated.

Solving problems using technology
In an attempt to ascertain whether people consider technology as a potential solution when they are trying to solve a problem, a hypothetical situation was presented to the focus groups in the form of a vignette. This first vignette described a situation that someone with memory loss might find him or her self in. It was used to find out how people might try to solve the problems described in the account.

George is a widower aged 78 years, who has lived in his own bungalow for five years. Since his wife died two years ago he has been living on his own. He has no close relatives. His home is large and difficult to heat. There is no gas supply to the house. He uses electric fires to heat his living room and his kitchen. George cooks for himself. He sometimes leaves the cooker and the fire full on in the kitchen when he returns to the lounge. George enjoys making his own meals. The neighbours are concerned about the risk of fire.

What could be done to help George? There are no right or wrong answers to this question.

Health and social care professionals suggested that *"in the early stages you could use signs to say remember to turn the cooker off"* (occupational therapist) or *"just a simple note [saying] remember to turn the cooker off"* (home care assistant). However if this intervention failed the most likely solution to be adopted would be the disconnection of the cooker, *"the cooker would be switched off and he would get meals delivered"* (social worker) *"the cooker is disconnected and meals on wheels are organised".* (care manager).

Professionals acknowledged that this solution would probably have a negative effect for the person with dementia, *"every kitchen has a cooker in it, it is part of our culture so removing it is a big thing"* (care manager) *"and those sort of things happen which are ultimately taking things away from the individual"* (social worker). Some suggested a preferred solution: *"in an ideal world someone with him at lunchtime to work with him".* (social worker).

Carers and people with dementia also indicated that they felt it was important to support him to continue to cook *"(it's...) quality of life we are talking about aren't we - maintaining quality of life"* (ex-carer) *"somebody could come round and check on him".* (person with dementia) One fear was that the perceived risk might result in the person having to leave their home, *"move him".* (person with dementia)

Both groups made suggestions on how the problem might be solved using existing technological devices. This included the use of smoke alarms, fire blankets, cooker guards and safer forms of heating such as storage heaters and oil filled radiators.

The use of a timer on the cooker was also suggested but there was uncertainty as to whether a specific timer was manufactured for use with electric cookers.

In addition HIA and DIY staff made suggestions concerning potential adaptations which could be made to the cooker but these were qualified with the following statement *"any problem like this is that you are now doing a modification to a piece of electrical equipment and it falls into all sorts of rules. You can't just rewire cookers"* (DIY retailer)

Ethical dilemmas
In an attempt to ascertain how people make decisions relating to 'whose choice it is to use technology' the second vignette was introduced to the focus groups. This presented an ethical dilemma in an attempt to explore how people 'hear the voice' of the person with dementia.

Mrs Jones lives alone in a council flat. She is well known and liked locally. Her daughter lives locally and visits regularly. She has good neighbours. Sometimes she gets up in the middle of the night and goes out into the street. This causes a great deal of worry for her family and her neighbours. The local authority has offered to fit an alarm on her front door, which would operate on a timer. If she went out between 10pm and 7am the alarm would be raised at a local 'Life line centre' and her family could be alerted. The fitting of the alarm has been discussed with Mrs Jones but she does not want it to be fitted.

(Based on case study reported by Marshall 2001)

What could be done to solve this problem? Once again there are no right or wrong answers to this question.

Health and social care professionals said that the most important factor for them in making a decision would be identifying the 'actual' level of risk to the person with memory loss as opposed to the 'perceived' level of risk: *"I think you need to look at the risk: how often is she wandering, does she return by herself, is she appropriately dressed when she goes out - those sort of things"* (community psychiatric nurse). *"Family sometimes feel guilty and over react to danger"* (occupational therapist). *"People are naturally paternalistic about people but you just tell them that you know what the risks are and you have minimised them"* (care manager).

Professionals also recognised that other issues may sometimes need to be addressed before using an alarm. *"The reason that she is getting up at night may be that she is disorientated so that needs to be addressed"* (care professional). *"Looking at her day routine is she being stimulated enough or is she sleeping during the day so that she is awake at night"* (care manager). *"Why is she waking up at night and going out? Does her medication need to be looked at?"* (community psychiatric nurse).

They also suggested that they would look for alternative solutions to the problem. *"You could look at alternatives. There could be something else, like a little note on the door or something"* (care manager). *"Maybe it would be just a matter of fixing a talking clock to the door then she*

might realise that it is the middle of the night and not the middle of the day" (care professional). *"Some sort of tracking device would be helpful"* (home care assistant).

Some people suggested that providing an example of how the device worked might support the person with dementia to make an informed choice as to whether or not to have the alarm fitted: *"Perhaps she doesn't really understand what it is all about perhaps if she could be taken to somebody who has got one to give her an insight"* (carer). *"See if she would be agreeable to trying it for a week on a trial basis with a clear understanding that it would be removed unless she actually says, well, I would like it to stay so she's actually got the choice. She is more able to make an informed choice that way because she's actually had some idea of what it is like"* (care manager).

Persuasion was also discussed as a method of getting the person with memory loss to accept the installation of the alarm: *"Saying to her that all other options have been exhausted, people are worried and would you consider trying it to be able to stay in this flat"* (care manager). *"Sit down with her and try and discuss it further and say how beneficial it would be for her and give her family peace of mind"* (home care assistant). *"She would have to be reasoned with. The daughter would really have to get on and say look mum unless you allow us to do this you will have to go into a home"* (ex-carer).

Opinions varied as to whose responsibility it would be to persuade the person with memory problems to accept installation of the alarm: *"It would be better to use the family to try and persuade her I certainly wouldn't want to be enforcing something like that on her"* (care professional). *"The ideal situation for you is to find out who she trusts whether it's her doctor or a neighbour or someone like that. Let them try and persuade her - someone she will listen to"* (ex-carer).

Some felt that if the perceived level of risk necessitated it they would resort to fitting the alarm without the knowledge of the person with memory loss. *"I mean I can't see why they couldn't have the alarm put in - take her out for the day somewhere and have the alarm put in and she wouldn't know anything about it"* (carer). *"I think if all else fails you have to have it fitted where they can't see it"* (ex carer). *"You are being underhand but you have to do it"* (carer). *"If she is not aware that it is there then that would be okay"* (carer).

Concern for the amount of stress that neighbours might experience was also responsible for the decision of some carers to fit the alarm. *"Anything could happen. It's not fair on the neighbours"* (carer). *"There are other people involved. There is family. They are entitled to live a life without worrying so are the neighbours....... so it is not just about her although it is her right to have or not to have something. There are other people as far as I am concerned.... do it* (fit the alarm) *and never mention it again to her"* (HIA member of staff).

The question of human rights was also considered. Some felt that it would be *"going against her human rights"* (occupational therapist). *"I think it is an intrusion into her privacy really and I don't think we have any right to go and put something in that she disagrees with"* (carer). *"I would be very wary of doing that* (fitting the alarm without her knowledge) *knowing*

that Mrs Jones didn't want it" (HIA member of staff).

Others however felt that safety came before human rights, *"I would fit it because I mean human rights are alright but it is for her own benefit"* and *"that's common sense (fitting alarm without the person knowing) but they will say that she has got human rights"* (female carer).

The responses to the story portrayed in the vignette illustrate the ethical dilemmas and conflicts surrounding the use of technology. Ethical concerns need to be approached constructively, considered and addressed (Cash 2003). As Marshall (1997) cautions, we need 'to be open and honest' about why we use technology. We need to ensure that technology is being used to meet the needs of the person with dementia in an 'empowering and enabling way' (Gilliard 2001), it is no longer acceptable to justify the use of technology solely using the principle of beneficence.

Comprehensive guidance for health and social care professionals on addressing ethical issues relating to the use of technology is provided in both the ASTRID guide (Marshall 2000) and the TED (Technology, Ethics and Dementia) guidebook (Bjørneby *et al* 1999).

Phase 2.

People recruited
A total of 31 people were referred to the project and of these 28 trialled devices. Two failed to give consent and one person was admitted to hospital prior to the consent procedure. Their ages ranged from 63-89 years. Just over half (57%) lived alone and the remainder lived with a spouse. Over a quarter (28%) lived in warden

assisted accommodation. Two participants living in warden-assisted accommodation were unable to nominate carers.

Devices

Participants were invited to select one device from those identified which best matched their individual need.

i. Locator device

The locator device is aimed at enabling people to locate items, which they frequently misplace. The device has four colour-coded buttons (red, yellow, blue and green) each of which has space next to the button for a picture or the name of the object to be located. Four tags whose colours correspond with the buttons on the locator unit can be attached to items by means of a key ring or a Velcro tab. When the user touches a button it initiates a bleeping sound from the tag attached to the misplaced item so that it can be found. The sound stops when the item is picked up.

Implementation

The device comes with a base unit that has a magnetic strip for attachment purposes (the device can be used without this unit). The locator device is battery operated. The items, which are frequently misplaced, need to be identified and tagged accordingly. It is important that the locator unit is kept in a location that is familiar to the user. It is necessary to check that the user can hear the sound and recognize that it is coming from the tag attached to the misplaced object. If the user lives alone they require the ability to learn new routines, as they have to understand how to operate the device.

Reliability of product

No technical problems were reported with the product. Clear operating instructions were provided by the manufacturers and these were given to the participants and their carers.

Case example.
Nancy, aged 83 years, lives alone. She has home care and is also supported by a neighbour. She attends a day centre on several days a week. Nancy's handbag is a very important to her and she likes to have it with her at all times in particular when she attends the day centre. Nancy frequently misplaces her handbag and if her neighbour is unable to find it she gets very distressed. This is a particular problem on the days she attends the day centre, as she will not leave home without it. Nancy agreed to try a locator device. Although Nancy was not able to operate the device herself her neighbour was able to locate the handbag using the device and involved Nancy in listening for the bleep from the tag. Nancy no longer worries about misplacing her handbag, as she is confident that her neighbour will be able to locate it for her. Nancy is now able to attend the day centre regularly.

Suggestions for improvement

People were asked how they thought the product could be improved. The most common comment was that, *"the bleep is not very loud. If you are looking for modifications that is something. You could make the bleep a bit louder"* (carer). The size of the tags was also commented on. Some people found that their size restricted them from tagging some items that they frequently misplaced like spectacles and hearing aids. People who used the Velcro pads to attach the tags to items commented that they had problems making them adhere, *"Maybe not strong enough or not sticky enough"* (carer).

The locator device was the most popular device and was used by 12 participants suggesting that misplacing items is of concern to both people with dementia and their carers. The device was most successful where there was a carer to support its use. One person managed to operate the device following instructions from her son over the telephone.

"On the telephone and I would ask her to go and press the button and locate it. It gives me more confidence that things at a distance are under control, because I know that it is possible to locate something in a different way from just talking it through, because mum has been as long as perhaps three quarters of an hour looking for her medication in the past" (carer).

The most commonly tagged items were keys and handbags. The most unusual item tagged was a tortoise!

Comments from those who used the locator device

Time saving
"Saving time and worry really because it's important if you mislay the keys" (carer). *"Normally we would be looking absolutely everywhere every drawer every cupboard, wardrobe, washing basket we would have to empty everything out just to find it"* (non-resident carer).

Relieving stress
"I've stopped worrying about where to find the keys because I know now I can find them and I don't have to worry" (carer). *"It's stopped me getting bad*

tempered" (carer) *"Yes it's saved us aggro"* (carer).

Reducing the need to invade privacy
"It is much easier. It stops me having to rifle through all the drawers and cupboards which people find very offensive, people don't like you going through their personal belongings" (home care assistant).

Professionals views about the value of the device
Professionals indicated that the device provides support for both the person with dementia and those who care for them.

	Yes	No/no difference	n/k or missing
Increased contact with client	2 (17%)	5 (42%)	5 (42%)
Provided support for client	6 (50%)	1 (8%)	5 (42%)
Provided support for carer	6 (50%)	0	6 (50%)
Increased the amount of time the person with dementia lived at home	1 (8%)	2 (17%)	9 (75%)

Table 2. Professional's evaluation of the usefulness of the locator device

Table 2 provides a breakdown of the views of professionals about the usefulness of the locator device. Though the majority did not think it had led to any increase in contact with the client, half thought that it had provided support for the person with dementia and carer respectively.

ii. Medication reminder

The purpose of the medication reminder is to dispense the correct medication at the correct time. The reminder is a circular container with a lockable lid. Inside the container is a rotating cassette, which has twenty-eight compartments into which the medication is dispensed. This allows pills to be dispensed up to four times a day. At pre-programmed times the cassette rotates, an alarm signal sounds and the correct dosage of medication comes into view through an opening in the lid. Tilting the reminder dispenses the medication; this allows the medication to fall into the hand of the person using it. This action stops the alarm. If the person fails to carry out this action the alarm will continue to ring for approximately 25 minutes. If the medication is not removed when the dose is due the action of the carousel rotating results in the missed medication being retained inside the container.

Implementation

An instruction booklet is provided with the device. The reminder needs to be programmed with the times that the medication is due to be taken. It also requires someone to dispense the medication in the correct doses into the reminder. In some cases a carer performed these tasks. If a carer was unable to undertake these tasks it required the support of a pharmacist. The device is battery operated and it requires someone to take responsibility for changing the batteries. This could be a potential problem if a pharmacist is dispensing medication into the reminder, as someone would need to take responsibility for the purchase of the batteries. It is also necessary for the alarm to be re-programmed to take account for seasonal time changes. Seven people volunteered to use this device.

Reliability

The alarm was reported as going off at the set times. One person identified a problem with a tablet getting stuck between the opening and the lid on one occasion. Some people found the lock difficult to open.

Case example.
Paul lives alone. His wife died recently. Whilst she was alive she reminded him to take his medication. Since her death his son who lives a long way away has taken responsibility for reminding his father by telephoning him twice a day. This is not always convenient for him as he works irregular hours. The son programmed the reminder for his father. Paul finds the reminder easy to use and is pleased to be able to take responsibility for taking his medication. His son no longer has the burden of remembering to telephone his father twice a day at set times.

Suggestions for improvements

The most frequent suggestion for improvement made by carers was that the low battery indicator should be visible from the outside of the reminder. Some also felt that it would be helpful if the lid could be made from a semi-transparent material to enable them to check if any medication has not been taken and to monitor the timer clock. One person felt it would be useful to have simple operating instructions printed on the bottom of the reminder in case the instruction booklet was mislaid or lost.

Comments from those who used the medication reminder

Compensating for impaired memory

"Oh quite easy yes, it goes off like an alarm clock does, and then it produces the tablets. You can't get the tablets without, without it goes off you know, yes it's been working alright" (person with dementia). *"Well oh yes I think it is very clever but when I first got I thought why don't they let me have three bottles and I'll remember to take*

them" (person with dementia). "*I would be lost without it*" (person with dementia). "*If I didn't have this machine I wouldn't be taking them I would completely forget and I wouldn't remember if I had taken them or not*" (person with dementia).

Support for carers
"*To know that she is actually taking them you know regularly*" (female non-resident carer).

"*I can come at the end of the week and open it up and see exactly what she has taken and what she hasn't taken and I know exactly what is going on*" (male non-resident carer).

"*It's made it a lot easier because I know my dad is getting the medication that he needs*" (male non-resident carer).

"*Peace of mind I suppose really at the end of the day*" (male non-resident carer).

Professionals views about the value of the device
Professionals indicated that the device provides support for both the person with dementia and their carers.

Table 3 provides a breakdown of the views of professionals about the usefulness of the medication reminder. Over half thought that the device had increased the amount of time that the person with dementia lived at home.

	Yes	No/no difference	n/k or missing
Increased contact with client	0	4 (57%)	3 (43%)
Provided support for client	5 (71%)		2 (29%)
Provided support for carer	3 (43%)		4 (57%)
Increased the amount of time the person with dementia lived at home	4 (57%)		3 (43%)

Table 3. Professional's evaluation of the usefulness of the medication reminder

The majority of professionals felt that the medication reminder helped to support both the person with dementia and their carer.

iii. Memo minder

The Memo minder is a message recorder/player operated by battery or AC adaptor. A message of up to 20 seconds in length can be recorded onto a circuit board. The message is triggered by a passive infra-red motion detector whenever anyone moves within a range of 5 metres or 15 degrees of the memo minder.

Implementation
An instruction manual is provided with this device. The chosen message is recorded on the device by sliding the function switch to the 'REC' position and then depressing the 'REC/PLAY' button until the recording is completed. The message is erased if you start to record a new message. The device can be placed on a table/shelf or mounted on a wall. It is important to locate the device in a position where the message can be activated by the movement of the user. If the message only needs to be played at certain times of the day or night it requires someone

to switch the memo minder on and off at appropriate times.

The nature of the message recorded on the memo minder depended on the individual need of the users. In all cases the person recording the message was known to the user; so the voice they heard giving the message was familiar to them.

The following reminders were recorded:
- To remember to lock the door and take the keys with them when they were going out;
- Not to go out during the night (2);
- To wait until home care arrived before getting up in the morning;
- To indicate whether it was a day to attend the day centre;
- To indicate where the carer had gone and when they would be returning (this carer made use of the device's ability to record new messages).

Reliability of product
No problems were reported.

Case example.
James lives alone in sheltered housing. He attends a day centre on several days a week and he also likes to go out walking in the local neighbourhood. When he leaves his flat he forgets to lock his front door and often leaves the door open as well. Recently there have been a number of thefts in the area. Friends of James recorded a message reminding him to lock his door and take his keys with him when he goes out. James responds well to this reminder and locks his door when he goes out. He recognises that the voice belongs to a friend and says that he finds the voice reassuring.

Suggestions for improvement
The only suggestion for improvement was for the device to incorporate a timer so that it did not rely on someone to be available to turn it on and off at set times.

Comments from those who used the memo minder
"*Yes very helpful yes it puts my mind at rest sort of thing*" (person with dementia).
"*Were it to be absent I think I might forget so I am pleased to have it*" (person with dementia).
"*Very helpful sometimes I go out early and it says to stay in bed*" (person with dementia)

Support for carers
"*From the feedback that I have had or not had it must have been very useful because no-one has been complaining about early morning phone calls saying he is getting out of bed at four o'clock in the morning*" (home care assistant).

"*Prior to that I would have had a piece of paper and wrote down where I was going but when I come home it is in the bin and he's forgotten where I've been so this will keep repeating itself until I come in the front door and switch it off again and then it has given reassurance to know where I have gone which has been most useful*" (resident carer).

Negative comments
"*She became very agitated by being told what to do*" (non-resident carer).

"*I don't know boxes and noises. If you want to go you go*" (person with dementia).

Professionals views about the value of the device

Professionals again indicated that the device provided support for both the person with dementia and those who cared for them. Table 4 provides a breakdown of the views of professionals about the usefulness of the memo minder. In half of the cases they indicated that it had supported the person with dementia to continue living at home. The reminder appeared to work well for people with mild to moderate dementia. In the two cases where the device was not perceived as providing support the participants had more severe dementia and became intolerant of the voice and were annoyed by it.

	Yes	No/no difference	n/k or missing
Increased contact with client	0	6(100%)	
Provided support for client	4 (67%)	1(17%)	1(17%)
Provided support for carer	4 (67%)	1(17%)	1(17%)
Increased the amount of time the person with dementia lived at home	3 (50%)	2 (33%)	1(17%)

Table 4. Professional's evaluation of the usefulness of the Memo Minder.

The majority of professionals felt that the memo minder provided support to both the person with dementia and their carer.

iv. Telephone

The telephone identified in phase I of the research was a picture telephone. In addition to the normal keys this telephone had nine large pre-programmable keys, to which a photograph or the name of a person could be added. This allows the person to dial a number by pressing one key and eliminates the need to remember a string of numbers. However this telephone was not available during phase II of the project. A similar telephone was located but the pre-programmable buttons on this telephone only had space for a name to be written by the side of them.

Implementation

The existing telephone was replaced by the pre-programmable telephone. A family member programmed the required numbers and wrote the names by the side of the buttons. The person with dementia needs to be able to recognize the names written by the side of the buttons in order to identify the correct button to push.

Reliability

No problems were reported.

Suggestions for improvements

No suggestions were made.

Case example.
Rosemary lives with her husband. She has lost confidence in using the telephone because she is unable to remember telephone numbers and has subsequently stopped using the telephone. A family member programmed the telephone with the telephone numbers of her family and friends. Rosemary is gaining confidence in using a telephone again both to make and answer calls. She is now able to contact her family and friends and this is helping her to maintain her social network. She says that this has helped her to feel 'better about herself'.

Comments from those who used the telephone

"Well before I wouldn't use it, it has been very useful because before I didn't like to touch the phone...I just pick it up and press the button and

then you know I haven't got to worry" (person with dementia).

"You used to make a call and you would be half way through and then you'd forget the number" (resident carer).

Professional's evaluation of the device

The professional who made the referral was unable to comment on how successful the device had been as she had had no further contact with the person since making the referral.

v. Passive infra-red (PIR) night light

A number of lighting devices were identified in phase I of the research. These ranged from dusk to dawn lights which plug into an existing electrical socket and emit a low level light throughout the hours of darkness to hard wired light switches which react to either body heat or movement to activate a light which can be programmed to stay on for a set number of minutes. The person who elected to trial a night-light chose to use a dusk to dawn light, which had a PIR function.

Implementation

Two PIR dusk to dawn lights were used. One was plugged into an existing plug socket by the bed and the other was plugged into an existing plug socket in the hallway near to the toilet door. Both lights were switched to the PIR function so that they only came on when activated by movement. The lights stayed on for approximately one minute when activated. This enabled the person to see to find their way from the bedroom to the hallway and then to locate the toilet.

Reliability

No problems were reported.

Suggestions for improvement

No suggestions were made.

> **Case example.**
> **Joan and Peter live in a bungalow. Peter gets up during the night to use the toilet and sometimes becomes disorientated in the darkness. If he switches on the main lights this disturbs Joan's sleep and she finds it difficult to get back to sleep. PIR Night Lights come on when Peter gets out of bed and light the way to the toilet. This allows him to orientate himself and find the way to the toilet safely. Joan's sleep is now less disturbed.**

Comments from those who used the night light.

"I know where to go now, you get used to it, I know where to go" (person with dementia).

"Once you've got that main light on it wakes you up. I was awake for hours after" (female carer).

Professional's evaluation of the device

The professional who made the referral was unable to comment on how successful the device had been as she had had no further contact with the person since making the referral.

vi. Door alarm

A number of different door alarms were identified in Phase I of the project. The one trialled was a wire free PIR contact door alarm with a portable alarm unit. This alarm was selected to meet the individual needs of the people involved.

Implementation

This device requires someone to attach contact switches to the door and doorframe. The packaging contained installation instructions.

Reliability

Initially the alarm failed to work correctly after installation and made a constant beeping noise. This was due to a problem with the installation and not with the device itself.

Suggestions for improvement

No suggestions were made.

Case example.

Sarah & David live in a first floor maisonette. David has dementia. His wife Sarah is hearing impaired and has restricted mobility. David likes to go out walking. David is disorientated in time and is often away for long periods of time when he goes for a walk. This is a particular problem in the summer when the evenings are light. Sarah is often unaware that David has gone out because she is unable to hear the front door opening and closing. This causes Sarah to worry because she has no idea how long he has been absent from the house. The portable door alarm indicates to Sarah when David has left the house and when he returns. This provides re-assurance for her and allows her to decide if she needs to alert someone to look for David if he has been gone for a long period of time. David is able to maintain some independence by continuing with an activity he enjoys.

Comments from those who used the door alarm

"I thought the other day that it would make sense to ring every time I go out and you know I've gone out" (person with dementia).

"I know when my husband has gone out and I hear him come back. So I can relax and think right he is home" (carer).

Professionals views about the value of the device

The referring professional was of the opinion that the door alarm had offered support both to the person with dementia and the carer but that it did not appear to have made a difference to the level of contact the person with dementia experienced.

Discussion

Assistive devices

Results from the focus groups and semi-structured interviews suggest the task of identifying and locating appropriate devices can be a time consuming process. Some of the devices identified in phase I of the study were either no longer available for purchase - for example, the picture phone - or the original source of supply had changed by the time trials of devices commenced in phase II of the study.

Manufacturers may also be unaware of the potential of their products to support people with dementia. For example, the locator device is principally marketed as a 'gadget' and the picture phone was discontinued from the product range when the distributor of this product was taken over. A greater awareness of the problems facing people with dementia needs to be promoted amongst manufacturers to help them not only to design and supply products that would provide support, but to successfully market existing products that have potential to do so.

Installing assistive devices

Finding appropriately qualified and trained contractors to install devices was identified as a problem in the BESTA project. (Bjørneby, 2000). In this project only two devices required installation by someone other than a family carer. In both of these cases the participants were members of HIA schemes and the devices were fitted by members of their staff. In the case of the door alarm the agency had to arrange a return call because the alarm failed to function correctly after it was installed. This resulted in a delay of approximately two weeks before the alarm was fully functioning, because this was the earliest return appointment the agency could offer.

People with dementia may need support to find appropriately qualified contractors to install devices. Appropriate training for those involved in the installation of devices should be considered in order to enable them to work in a way that supports the needs of the person with dementia. Systems to secure this should be addressed by decision makers and could involve joint working between local authorities and HIA's.

The role of assistive technology in supporting people with dementia

This study has provided evidence that assistive technology devices can provide support to both people with dementia and carers. Evidence collected suggests that a range of factors may be involved in successful implementation.

For the person with dementia, successful use of technology: acceptance of having a memory problem, motivation to use the device, ability to learn new tasks if the device requires user input, the ability of someone to provide support in the initial stage of use and a positive relationship with their primary caregiver.

For the carer, success may depend on their willingness to support the person with dementia in their use of the device.

Wider social factors will also be important. The role, attitude and understanding of all health and social care and housing professionals involved with the person with dementia and their willingness to provide support in all aspects of using the device are likely to be very important. This will include sourcing devices, ensuring they are installed, work properly and meet the needs for which they are intended. Professionals will also have a central role in supporting the use of the device – for example arranging and agreeing any responses that may be needed when devices are activated and indicate that a response of some kind may be needed. Finally, they will also have a part to play in decommissioning the device when it no longer provides support or is no longer needed.

The characteristics of the devices themselves will also have some bearing on successful use. The reliability, aesthetics, ease of use, ease of installation, ease of maintenance and cost of the device are all likely to be significant.

There is a need for an assessment tool to be developed that takes the above factors into account. There is a need for more training to be available to health and social care professional, as well as those who work in housing and Home Improvement Agencies.

Conclusion

At Home with AT was an innovative study that investigated the ability of low technological devices to provide support to people with dementia. The benefits of this form of technology are that devices:

- are readily available for purchase;
- can be used in the existing home of the person with dementia;
- do not require the installation of sophisticated computer equipment;
- can be easily removed or adapted as the needs of the person with dementia change.

This study aimed to raise awareness at all levels of the potential of low-level technology to support people with dementia and carers. It has highlighted the need for more work to be done to promote and develop low-level assistive technology on a national scale.

References

Allan, K., (2001) Communication and Consultation: Exploring ways for staff to involve people with dementia in research. Policy Press, Bristol.

Bartlett, H., & Martin, W., (2002) *Ethical Issues in Dementia Care Research.* In Wilkinson, H., (ed.) The Perspectives of People with Dementia: Research methods and motivations. London, Jessica Kingsley.

Bjørneby, S., (2000) *'Smart Houses': Can They Really Benefit Older People?* Signpost, Vol. 5, No 2; 34-36.

Bjørneby, S., & van Berlo, A., (eds.) (1997) Ethical Issues in Use of Technology for Dementia Care. Netherlands, Akontes Publishing.

Bjørneby, S., Topo, P., & Holthe, T., (eds.) (1999) Technology, Ethics and Dementia. Norway, INFO-banken.

Cash, M., (2003) *Assistive Technology and People with Dementia.* Reviews in Clinical Gerontology 13: p. 313-319, Cambridge University Press.

Department of Health., (2000) *The NHS Plan - A Plan for Investment, a Plan for Reform.*

Department of Health., (2001a) *The National Service Framework for Older People.*

Department of Health (2001b) *The Integrated Community Equipment Services Initiative.*

Fisk, M.J., (2001) *The Implications of Smart Home Technologies.* In: Peace, S. M., & Holland, C., (eds.), Inclusive Housing in an Ageing Society - Innovative approaches. Bristol Policy Press, p.101-123.

Gilliard, J., (2001) *Technology in Practice: Issues and Implications,* Journal of Dementia Care; Jan - Feb: p. 28-31.

Marshall, M., (1997) *The Ethical Use of Ttechnology.* Care Plan, 4:11-13.

Marshall, M., (1999) *Person-Centred Technology.* Signpost; 3: p. 4-5.

Marshall, M., (ed.) (2000) ASTRID: A Social and Technological Response to meeting the needs of Individuals with Dementia and their carers: A guide to using technology within dementia care. London, Hawker.

Marshall, M., (2001) *Dementia and Technology.* In: Peace, S. M., & Holland, C., (eds.) Inclusive Housing in an Ageing Society - Innovative approaches. Bristol, Policy Press, p. 125-143.

Tinker, A., (2003) *AssistiveTechnology and its Role in Housing Policies for Older People.* Quality in Ageing- Policy Practice and Research. Pavilion Publishing; 4 August: p. 4-12.

3. Person Centred Approaches to Using Technology in Practice Settings: the South Lanarkshire Dementia Technology Initiative

Christine Calder, South Lanarkshire Social Work Department.

The South Lanarkshire Dementia Technology Initiative was set up to explore the potential of technology and its application with people with dementia and to make staying at home a real possibility for people with dementia. The project idea came from literature searches that were undertaken to establish if any other local authorities were involved in the use of assistive technology and the Technology Ethics and Dementia (*TED*) guidance (Bjørneby *et al.* 1997) provided the foundation from which the project was developed.

Teamwork and collaboration are central to promoting the most practical and effective solutions to meet the needs of people who contact providers of assistive technology services. Within South Lanarkshire an Interdisciplinary Team (Technology Clinic) was set up to progress referrals. It has proved to be a good way to deliver the service, bringing together experience from a variety of backgrounds, including social work, health, housing, and control centre staff. Locally based technology advisors within Social Work teams provide day to day advice on the range of equipment and its applicability. At the time of writing a technical team is just about to be brought on stream to undertake installations, routine checks, battery replacement, etc. This teamwork - in partnership with the technology clinics and the technology advisors - enables person-centred responses to equipment when activated. The technology advisors are based in local social work teams and are a mix of social workers, social work assistants and resource workers. Some had experience of working with people with dementia while others had a good working knowledge of the community alarm service and some of the associated technology. Technology awareness sessions were held for the advisors. These included an introduction to the range available, the use of the 10 step guide in the *TED* Guidance and the procedures for referrals, funding and ongoing support.

Initially the project was set up to offer technological support to ten people. Those recruited were nominated by their care managers. No diagnosis of dementia was required since the project management team was clear from the outset that that the project should be as 'inclusive' as possible. There was an awareness that staff were already supporting people with complex packages of care in the community who had significant cognitive impairment but with no diagnosis of dementia who would clearly benefit from the application of assistive technology. The team were also very aware of the stigma diagnosis can bring and the stress this can involve for the person and their family. It was felt that insisting on a diagnosis of dementia would have put too many people off from participating.

Six of the ten participants had already experienced 'wandering' from home or had difficulty in using domestic appliances properly resulting in fires and floods. The care managers and family/carers of those nominated were also committed to supporting the person's wishes to stay at home.

Care was taken to ensure that the use of any device was strictly controlled and did not impinge on individual human rights. Members of staff were advised through training that the use of technology had to be consistent with procedures and guidance developed for this purpose. Its use is also regularly reviewed by a senior officer in social work. The deployment of the technology also enhanced the service currently provided by the council via its community alarm service operated by their 24 hour control centre. In South Lanarkshire the Community Alarm Service is managed within the Housing & Technical Resources Department but the staff who respond to the alarm and technology activations are managed within the Social Work Department.

In order to ensure that the assessment for technology was person-centred, the decision was made not to develop forms or other paperwork to access equipment. Instead assessors were asked, as part of the community care assessment, to identify where technology might be applied and what the expectations would be, as part of the overall package of care. The assessment also had to list the other solutions that had been considered or tried out before arriving at the 'technology solution'. Consent was sought and recorded in the assessment. Staff were also encouraged to use the services of an advocacy worker where appropriate. If consent wasn't obtained this would be recorded in the assessment, as well further actions that may have been taken, and why.

Before supplying the technology, staff were asked to consider if the use of technology was person-centred and if a risk assessment had been undertaken. Questions about dignity and privacy were also asked.

A guide was produced and circulated to all social work staff. Alongside this a rolling programme of training entitled 'The ethical use of assistive technology' allowed staff to consider practical as well as technical solutions for people with dementia living in the community who were identified as being at risk. All referrals to the project were considered by the older people's services manager and the resource worker to ensure that ethical issues were considered and recorded. This often involved discussion between the referrer and the resource worker and in many of these cases avoided 'knee jerk' responses to risk by social work staff. During this process practical solutions were often identified and to date one of the most successful solutions to someone wandering from home during the night has been a curtain drawn across the front door in the evening which prevented them from going out for quite some time before even considering door monitoring solutions.

The use of assistive technology can raise practical, technical and ethical issues. When technology is being assessed for, the assessor must be clear about what the technology *can* and *can't* do to reduce dangerous situations faced by vulnerable individuals. Family and carers need to be advised of this from the outset. A balance needs to be found between the wish to ensure privacy and safety for the service user on the one hand, and a realistic view of potential risks for service users on the other. For example, it may be reported by neighbours - or health and social work staff - that a person with dementia has gone out of the house at night on several occasions. Technology can be fitted to the door of the house which will activate a call to the control centre or a carer in order that they can respond to this and return the person home quickly and safely. However, an understanding of the context of the behaviour is essential if technology is to be used appropriately. There may be a number of possible underlying reasons for wandering, and observed behaviour may actually occur very infrequently. For example, nocturnal wandering might be due to clocks being put forward or back. It may therefore be that what is observed is not actually 'wandering' behaviour, but disorientation due to this change in time. It is therefore important that assessors clarify what risk *actually* exists before installing assistive technology. A good way of doing this is for staff keep a record for a few weeks in order that they can see if a pattern is developing or if indeed it was a 'one off' episode. The actual level of risk may not justify its use but might provide appropriate monitoring and reassurance for the service user and carer. If wrongly used however, it may provide false reassurance and be a waste of resources.

The ten participants in the South Lanarkshire Dementia Technology Initiative were provided with a social alarm unit, which is a telephone, linked to a 24 hour response centre. Some were receiving this service for the first time and others had their old system upgraded. The range of technology available in addition to this was discussed with the service users/carers and where possible consent was sought from service users or their representatives. None of the participants withheld consent, and the services of an independent advocate (encouraged by project team members) were not requested in any of the cases as all involved including the participants intimated a willingness to 'trial' the equipment in the first instance.

Three of the participants in whom definite patterns of 'wandering' had been identified had magnetic door contacts installed while the remaining seven did not require these devices as there had been one off episodes of 'wandering' but no real pattern had been identified as posing a risk. All ten participants had previously burnt cooking pans, causing smoke or small fires and all were fitted with a smoke alarm linked to the 24hr control centre and heat extreme detectors fitted in the kitchen and or living room/bedroom depending on the risk identified. Flood detectors were also provided where needed.

Two case studies

Mr E. One service user, Mr E, lived in a tower block and liked to hand-wash his clothes in the kitchen sink. On several occasions he forgot to turn the tap off which resulted in flooding of his flat and also the flat of downstairs tenants. The introduction of the flood detectors assisted in resolving the issue of significant water damage to his flat and others in the block while also reducing the level of 'crisis' experienced by Mr E and his family each time a flooding occurred. He had been discharged from hospital due to the support available from assistive technology. While in hospital an assessment of his needs was undertaken and it was recommended that he should be referred for 24hr care. Mr E had indicated all along that he wanted to return home and his family were very supportive of this, but were concerned about the number of floods and fires he had at home prior to admission to hospital and that these type of events might increase due to reduction in his cognitive ability. The assistive technology really worked well for Mr E – however, a solution was not identified that could support his continued use of the gas cooker. Devices are available to shut off gas supplies however they can only work successfully if robust response procedures are in place. The management of gas has proven to be a challenge in that there are a range of devices available but often when they are applied it only highlights the person's vulnerability if a relative cannot offer a 'social response' and can cause panic among the wider community when gas suppliers are being called to attend to a person's home on a regular basis.

Mr S. Mr S was also discharged from hospital due to the support provided by the technology. He was also assessed as requiring 24 hr care but expressed a desire to return to his own home. A visit was made to the home which was badly in need of minor repairs e.g. floor boards repaired and carpets replaced to prevent trip hazards and make the house more habitable. Mr S was prone to falling and therefore all repairs had to be carried out prior to any technology being provided Mr S lived in a semi rural area and his son lived in the same street but at the opposite end. In most cases where technology was installed, unless otherwise requested all alarm signals generated by technology were sent to social work home care staff responders who work from a 24hr control centre. In Mr S's case his son asked if he could be the first contact for any equipment which was activated. In order to provide as timely a response as possible, all of the technology was call routed to his mobile phone. This allowed him to speak direct to his father and provide reassurance and also provided a quicker response than could be made by the homecare staff who would need to travel some distance to get to him. Mr S was also provided with a fall detector but monthly

monitoring of his equipment and care package highlighted that when he was receiving his personal care the detector often got in the way or was removed and it was forgotten to put it back on. We looked at this issue and asked Mr S if he wanted to continue with the fall detector and he said he was happy to do so. A fall detector belt was purchased which allowed Mr S to receive his personal care without the fall detector being removed. He continues to wear the belt with success.

For all of the participants, monthly call histories were produced by the 24hr control centre which provided the Management Group with a clear picture of all the activity generated by the equipment. In conjunction with care managers, the project was able to identify where participants needs were changing and amend care packages accordingly. (Though for Mr S, due to the call routing set up, there was no paper trail of his technology being activated and in this case it meant a monthly feedback being provided directly from his care manager).

At the time of writing, three of the participants did move on from their own homes eventually: one to sheltered housing and two into residential care. In all cases, the care manager felt that the technology assisted them to stay at home longer than had been previously expected.

A number of insights were accumulated over the life of the project.

- Technology is not a panacea but it can enable people to live at home longer than expected providing it is installed early enough so that service users can become familiar with it.

- Pre-installation training is essential for all involved in the care of the service user, in order that the equipment is doing the job it was installed to do.
- Although there is no charge for the devices installed, service users/carers should be advised that the cost of a local telephone call is incurred each time the device is activated.
- People cannot be forced to wear or use assistive technologies no matter how beneficial they are deemed by professionals.
- Robust maintenance routines, testing procedures and battery replacement systems are needed to ensure that technologies are working and their functionality and reliability has not been compromised by some external event.
- Regular monitoring of the equipment is essential in order that the person's needs continue to be met and that the changes are logged with the care manager.
- A database for tracking of equipment is essential to ensure the optimization of all technologies installed.
- Response procedures must be developed and in place in advance of installation of equipment in order to insure that all activations are given considered support.
- A local infrastructure would be needed to allow a project to become a mainstream service.
- Key support and maintenance staff are required to ensure long term sustainability of such a service. Ongoing research and publicity is required to keep staff up to date on present and future technologies.
- Ongoing tests and development of equipment will be essential to provide equipment to suit the changing needs and complexities of individuals.
- The project has shown that new technology aids and devices can help people live more independently at home for longer periods of time and offer real alternatives to residential and nursing care. This may eventually have an impact on the numbers of people in need of future institutional care.
- Although the introduction of new technology has proved a success in terms of benefits to the service user group, resource issues have been identified in relation to staffing and service costs.
- An analysis of the calls history for each client both before and after the introduction of new technology has identified an increase in alarm activations. While this can easily be absorbed within the system with a small number of clients, as in the pilot phase, were it to be introduced on a larger scale then it would directly affect two key staff groups:

Control Centre staff, through….

  o Increased call volumes;
  o Increased participation in programming of equipment prior to installation;
  o Database maintenance – equipment control, battery replacement monitoring;
  o Increased training and awareness requirement (both initial and refresher training) with need to adapt to new equipment when introduced.

Responders (staff who may be called upon to respond when

technology provides an alerting signal), through....

- o Increased attendance to client group due to higher call activity;
- o Increased training and awareness requirement (both initial and refresher training) with need to adapt to new equipment when introduced;
- o Increased complexity in routine testing of peripheral equipment due to the location of sensors and nature of test procedure.

Technology can only be a supplement to meet the needs of people with dementia, and must always be used in the social context. When we discuss technology, we can think of very complex and sophisticated systems, or simple adaptations of households and all kinds of ordinary products and environments.

The South Lanarkshire Dementia Technology Initiative aimed to provide person-centred assistive technology applications and from current evidence we feel that this has been successful. Success depended upon clear guidance and procedures being in place for staff to follow and the whole approach of person-centred care must be the philosophy from which we work. The small number of participants allowed for the close monitoring and reviewing of the packages of care and the workers and carers and users commitment to the technology made it the success that it is. A risk, if a mainstream service were to be created would be that without the same commitment and enthusiasm they may not be as 'person-centred'.

Our increasing understanding of the experiences of people with dementia and their carers is encouraging the emergence of new approaches to care. Assistive Technologies have an important place in this new range of solutions. These developments are supporting a more positive approach to dementia care and the care of older people, where the aims are to improve quality of life, reduce risk, and encourage independence and to provide people with some real choices about remaining in their own homes.

Future plans include making proposals for the initiative to make the transition from project to mainstream service.

The technology advisors and representatives who made up the membership of the technology clinic were involved in other duties. A dedicated team is needed in order that staff can be provided with quicker access to advice and installation than at present.

Further funding options are being explored to allow the service to develop further in to using technology to support a wider range of people in the community and not just people with dementia or cognitive impairment.

Using technology to support carers in their caring role will also be another focus of the developing service.

References

Bjørneby, S., Topo, P., & Holthe, T., (1999) Technology, Ethics and Dementia, Norwegian Centre for Research on Dementia.

4. Creating the Building Blocks for an Integrated Technology Service - setting up the S.T.I.L. project in Norfolk

Dyllis Faife, Norfolk Social Services

My first real introduction to Assistive Technology was a visit to Northamptonshire Safe at Home Project's demonstration house in Northampton in May 2001. This feels like a very long time ago, and it was indeed a long and slow process before we were able to set up a Smart House in Norwich in March 2003. This illustrates the length of time it can take between having the seed of an idea, and actually achieving the end result. Since then, a change in the climate nationally and strong government support for developments in Assistive Technology means that progress will be much more rapid in the future.

With Central Government policy driving this agenda forward, backed up by the announcement of an £80 million Technology Prevention Grant for 2006-08, it should be possible for anyone wishing to set up a Smart Home Project - and to develop a technology based assessment service - to achieve this objective much more speedily and easily.

During the course of this article, my intention is to set out a first person account of where we are in Norfolk at the time of writing, how we have arrived there, what we are aiming for in the future, and how we are planning to get there. Hopefully the experience we have gained, and the lessons learned, will help others to achieve their objectives and may save them some time and energy along the way.

Overcoming obstacles

Partnership is key. I made two visits to the Smart Home in Northampton with different sets of colleagues from the partner agencies – a community mental health nurse, a consultant psychiatrist, an occupational therapist, the community alarms service manager and a housing support worker. I chose these particular colleagues as I was clear that the initial project which I wanted to set up should focus on supporting people with dementia (and their carers) to help them remain living at home, in a similar way as the Northampton Project. I believed that if we could solve the problems and overcome the challenges in supporting people with cognitive impairment, then supporting people with other physical health needs would be relatively easy.

My first visit to the Northampton demonstration house had really inspired me and it seemed to be an essential resource. For me, personally, there had been great benefit in actually 'seeing' the equipment in an ordinary domestic setting, and being shown how it worked, in order to understand and grasp the potential application of it, particularly as I am not a technologically sophisticated person. This view of the importance of 'seeing' it for oneself, as it was very new and 'different', was confirmed on the return from my first visit, when I wrote a paper about it for my department and it simply fell on stony ground. Another of my mad ideas. Words alone were not enough to convince people. So I quietly beavered on, and about a year later, made the second visit to Northampton, but this time with a really key colleague – the Community Alarms Service Manager, who worked for Norwich City Council. More of this later.

Project development requires a particular kind of person. Many years of project development has confirmed my view, that it is essential to have the right kind of colleagues with the right kind of approach – this makes all the difference between success and failure. Developing this particular project has reinforced that view. The kind of people you need are those with an entrepreneurial spirit. They have commitment, energy, and can grasp a new idea quickly, are keen and excited to go with it, prepared to take some risks, enjoy working in partnership, and are able to be flexible and innovative and prepared to share their resources. If you can find those qualities in a few colleagues, then you are at least half way there. It is also important to recognise that the qualities required for *project development* and the people that have them, will *not* be the same qualities and the same people you will need to approach for the *strategic development* of a totally integrated service across a wider geographical area.

Unless you are in the fortunate position of being ready to tackle the development of an assistive technology service from a strategic position straightaway – which may now be much more possible as the health and social care culture has shifted – our experience would suggest it may be better to start off with a small scale project. This provides the opportunity to develop protocols and procedures, and iron out any problems along the way.

Think of a good catchy name for your new project. Preferably one that can be reduced to a memorable acronym. We called our project the S.T.I.L at Home Project. This stands for *Supportive Technology for Independent Living at Home Project* and in the abbreviated title we can convey the overall essence of the project – which is about helping people to remain living at home. Our project has two parts to it – the establishment of a demonstration Smart House, and a related assessment project for people with dementia.

To have a Smart House, you need a building. We developed our first Norfolk Smart House in Norwich – finding a building is an early test of the effectiveness of partnership working. One of those invited to visit the demonstration house in Northampton – a colleague from Norwich City Council, was able to persuade the Council to provide us with a flat in a Sheltered Housing Scheme, from which existing tenants were being relocated. This meant vacant properties. We may need to move our current location within the next few months as the site is to be developed, but the current Smart House has served its purpose brilliantly. Since its inception in March 2003, well over two hundred and fifty people have visited our Smart House, including many professional staff from a variety of statutory agencies and voluntary organisations, carers groups and potential service users. It has proved to be an excellent resource for the whole of Norfolk. The Smart House does not have to be in a vacant Local Authority building – our next one will make use of an existing Sheltered Housing Scheme, but it could be in any appropriate building owned by any of the partners – for example it could be in an empty hospital ward.

We thought it was important to formally launch the project and involving the Sheriff of Norwich ensured that we received good publicity. Positive involvement of the media is important. During the last year, both our local MPs made formal visits to the Smart House. One of them is the Chair of the Science and Technology Committee, and one of them at the time of writing is the current Home Secretary, so we hoped that they would help us spread our message to higher places. Both were very enthusiastic and supportive, so the next lesson is to try and engage your local MP's or councillors.

The 'fame' of the Norwich Smart House has spread and we have received a number of visits by colleagues, from the Eastern Region particularly, and further afield, who are now looking to set up their own projects. We have been able to share our learning with them and hopefully help to speed up their projects.

The Smart House serves as a focus for the project. It is important to have clarity of purpose about any development and in my view the purpose of the Smart House is threefold: awareness raising, providing information, and education for service users, carers and professional staff. The issue of staff training is something which I will touch on later.

So, what else was needed to establish a Smart House? Well, the City Council donated the flat, we contacted local businesses to sponsor the furnishings (such as beds, carpets, chairs – as we wanted the environment to look like a real home), and we made contact with Tunstall Plc, who were able to provide most of the equipment without charge. Additional pieces of equipment were purchased by using Health and Social Care Award money (awarded for a different project in 2002) and this also initially financed the equipment required for individual people following assessment. The award money was actually a very small amount – only £2000, but the next part of my message would be that you don't have to have huge amounts of money, to start off such a project. You can be creative and innovative with small amounts of money, and use a small-scale 'pilot' project as the driver to take things forward. Working in partnership allows everyone to benefit from access to additional resources, and using the word 'pilot' allows flexibility, the opportunity to take risks and to try things out together, without needing to have that formal 'service level agreement'.

The pilot project was initially set up for two years, but after 1 year was already proving pivotal in driving forward the strategic agenda for developing an Assistive Technology service across Norfolk.

What is actually in the smart house?

We now have the following pieces of equipment installed, all of which link through to Community Alarm Service, mostly by the use of Radio Output modules:

- bogus caller button
- super smoke detector
- carbon monoxide detector
- gas detector with automatic shut-off valve
- flood detector
- temperature extremes detector
- falls detector
- bed-leaving monitor pressure mat / linked to lighting system
- door sensor 'wandering' device;
- PIR sensor movement detector.

Items such as the smoke detector can also be linked to a vibrating pillow or a flashing strobe light for people with visual impairment.

Much of the equipment we have used is provided by Tunstall PLC, but a number of other companies also provide similar equipment

These pieces of equipment operate as one part of a three part process:

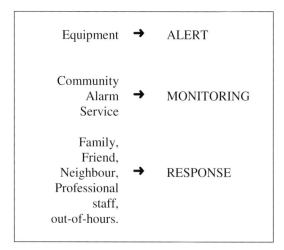

All elements are equally essential, and I will include more about the importance of the response later in the article, when I describe the assessment project.

As this project has specifically focused on supporting people with dementia, we also demonstrate additional pieces of stand-alone equipment:

- memo-minder
- locator device
- medication carousel
- electronic calendar
- day-date, am-pm office calendar.

We are always trying to check out which new pieces of equipment are available, but finding the time to do this is a real issue.

As an additional part of the overall project, we are also piloting the use of a 'prompting service', which is provided by the operators at the Community Alarms Service. This is a small-scale project, with up to about 10 to 12 people at any time. The social workers can send through information to request the type of prompt they require, such as medication reminder or day care reminder, and the operators make a manual contact over the telephone, to the service user, at the desired time and frequency. As well as the actual prompt itself, this operator service provides an extra form of social contact and thus the 'added value' of an informal befriending service.

Establishing a steering group.

It is really essential to establish a steering group if you are developing a project – our steering group has expanded and evolved, but I think our current representation is a fairly good model for others to consider. As the current project is dementia specific, the steering group has relevant membership, but these could be replaced by others, or added to, according to the actual remit of the project.

- Project co-ordinator
- community alarm service manager
- installation engineer
- social services representatives / social workers
- community mental health nurse
- occupational therapist
- housing support worker (more about this role later)
- Alzheimer's Society
- Care and Repair / Home Improvement Agency.

The group meets approximately monthly and the sharing of expertise has been extremely useful. A further key member is the minute taker – as without this extra ingredient I found I never actually had the time to write up any notes (and therefore no check on who hadn't followed up on the actions they were supposed to).

The assessment project

Having established the Smart House, a lot of creative energy was spent on coming up with 'just the right name' for the project. After that it was time to get down to the basics of the actual assessment and service delivery part of the project. As with any new service or project, the dissemination of information and communication is vital - and so we devised the S.T.I.L at Home Project leaflet. This describes the aims of the project and the referral procedure along with contact names. The leaflets were widely distributed to appropriate staff.

In order to help evaluate the project, one of the initial referral criteria was that each person should have a formal diagnosis of dementia. (However during the course of the project this particular criteria was relaxed as it became apparent that we might be excluding a number of people who could potentially benefit from this form of support). Referrals were accepted from social workers and community mental health nurses. We devised clear and simple criteria, referral forms, a descriptive equipment list for staff and review forms.

My experience has taught me that any new project does take time to establish itself, and not to expect referrals to come flooding in during the first few months. In fact, it usually seems to take about a year for any new project or service to become embedded in the psyche of very busy assessment staff. The S.T.I.L at Home Project has been no exception. During the second year, we have seen a significant increase in referrals. In addition, although *we* in the project team had already been convinced of the potential value of using assistive technology, for others, using technology to support people

still had the sense of something very new and rather strange about it. This wariness to engage in something new seemed even more apparent in relation to this project than in relation to other innovative service developments. It was important to recognise these concerns which the use of technology particularly elicited in people: that traditional anxiety about technology as 'big brother'.

During the course of the last two years, it has become apparent to me that what is still considered 'new' by health and social care staff (the technology itself) is considered very much 'old hat' by Housing colleagues. They are just wondering why we have all taken such a long time to catch up, when the potential application of assistive technology in terms of supporting people, has been obvious to them for quite some time.

Being aware of both how busy assessment staff are and taking account of their expressed concerns about technology, a model of service delivery was developed which assists their assessment role. This is achieved by involving existing housing support worker staff, who already provide an integrated service to both social workers and community mental health nurses in Norwich. The housing support workers are a small (3) key group of specialist staff, who take referrals from both professional groups and provide an intensive, short term service aimed at supporting older people with mental health needs to remain living in their own home. This is done by helping to promote independence and by helping people to achieve and regain their confidence and optimum ability.

The model is successful because it facilitates the role of the assessment staff and thereby encourages them to refer their clients to the project. The social workers and community mental health nurses were already confident about referring to this small, non-professionally qualified team who have much expertise, and their involvement with the technology project was simply an extension of this confidence. This team have now developed to become the 'experts', in terms of their increased knowledge of assistive technology, and understanding of its application, and they have the time to spend with clients and carers to inform and reassure them. They also undertake the reviews.

One of the housing support workers also now has the key task of showing visitors around the Smart House and demonstrating the equipment as a core part of the role.

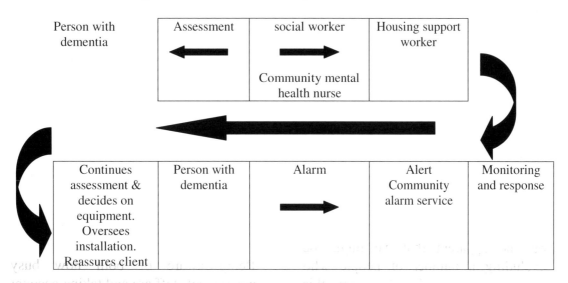

The project seems to have been very successful, although lack of time has limited me from collating the information collected in to a formal evaluation document as yet. Since April 2003 we have received 89 referrals for the assistive technology project for people with dementia. Most people have required only one piece of equipment, some have had two pieces and a very few, three pieces.

I am very clear that technology itself or indeed any one piece of technology does not 'fit all' – for some people with dementia, none of the technology is suitable, as it depends on how their dementia actually impacts on their daily life and the life of their carers. The assessment and assessment skills are still the *essential* aspect and overall key to the success of the project – the technology is merely one more tool, in the assessor's tool kit.

Other essential ingredients.

So far I have only briefly talked about installation. The basic community alarm equipment continues to be installed by the usual staff, but it is important to acknowledge the key contribution made by the Senior Installation Engineer, who has brought his own commitment and energy to the project – has grasped the potential, shared in the vision and helped to make it so successful using a creative approach to problem solving. Having the expertise of someone with the knowledge of electrical and gas installations has proved invaluable, and a prime example of the 'added value' of partnership and multi-disciplinary working. It has certainly not been traditional practice in Social Services to seek the opinions and perspective of an electrician when trying to solve the problem of how to support someone with dementia at home!

Following the assessments, many of the solutions, whilst still involving technology, have not involved the more complex monitoring by the community alarm service – but simple creative solutions. An example of this has been a carer, who has wanted to undertake the monitoring role, and where we installed a bed leaving pressure mat which, as well as being linked to bedside lighting and/or hardwired lighting, was also linked to a bell or buzzer in the separate bedroom where the carer slept.

Whilst creative energy is an essential ingredient to get things going, funding is the essential ingredient required to keep things going. In terms of project funding, I have adopted what I call the 'Haphazard Approach' or 'Seizing the Opportunity', and this in turn has led to opportunities to influence and begin to deliver a more strategically planned service.

Though at the start the project was funded with award money, once this was spent, and minds had been won over, we were able to move to using the Social Services 'Purchase of Care' budgets. These budgets are now being used to purchase the assistive technology equipment and to fund the installation costs as an alternative to the more traditional use of purchasing domiciliary and residential care. Service users continue to pay the basic community alarm rental charge in the usual way.

As the success of the Norwich based project has grown, so other colleagues around the county have slowly begun to access to project and spend their 'Purchase of Care' budgets on the service. For those situations where people may not meet the criteria for funding from these particular budgets, but have a carer who would benefit, then there is the possibility of accessing the carers' grant for a 'one-off' direct payment for carers, providing the criteria are met. Alternatively, people can decide to purchase the additional equipment and fund the installation privately, and then pay the ongoing Community Alarm service rental charge for the basic system and monitoring. Finally, as with other requests for assistance, charitable sources can always be approached.

As part of the next stage of my 'haphazard approach', the opportunity of European money was seized and after some 'fishing', I was made aware of a particular funding source, for developments in rural areas.

A successful application was made and we now have a small amount of funding over three years to develop the assistive technology service in the rural areas of Norfolk. This project has now commenced and will include establishing a Smart House in a market town serving the rural area, and a rural based dementia support project, based on our urban model. The European money will act as pump priming money to initiate the development of various rural projects around the county.

In trying to look at opportunities for this particular service development in as wide a context as possible, it has been possible to link assistive technology to a key government initiative of workforce redesign – this is about determining what kinds of staff, with what kinds of competencies, in what kinds of roles we need for the future to support those needing health and social care. Our bid to develop the service by creating new staff roles which will work across agencies, has been successful, and we will receive one year funding from TOPSS to begin to develop a county wide service during 2005-2006. These new roles, Assistive Technology Support Workers, will offer high levels of knowledge and skills in technology and a range of assessment skills. They will be pivotal in driving the service forward and developing partnership working, not only between Health and Social Care but also with Housing, Community Alarm Services and Home Improvement Agencies.

The strategic approach

To date, the Social Services Department and Social Services funding has been the driving force behind the developments in assistive technology in Norfolk. However, a unilateral approach can only achieve so much, now is the time to develop a more multi-lateral approach and Health Trusts in particular are likely to be key beneficiaries of a successful service. Within Norfolk, the Supporting People Commissioning Board agreed to inject funding during the next financial year via the Home Improvement Agencies to enable a more universal approach to the county wide development of the service. Funding would enable us to offer lower level preventative support and will operate in parallel to the TOPSS funding which will be used for targeting the more vulnerable people with a higher level of need. So, one open door was intended to stimulate another door to open. (Unfortunately, the Supporting People Team later decided that this proposal would not meet their criteria and was withdrawn. Discussions continue to try and find a resolution as to how best to fund low

level preventive technology support, as this is such an important area of out work).

At the beginning of this article I said that those who need to be engaged in the strategic development and delivery of the service are likely to be different people to those who helped to set up the project. The major motivating forces in their working lives will be the achievement of targets, service delivery plans and performance indicators.

They will not necessarily have the vision and commitment of those initially involved but they will hold the 'purse strings' and be the access route to delivering the vision strategically. There are numerous agencies and bodies which have an interest in developing an Assistive Technology service (see the attached diagram) – it's just that some of them haven't quite realised it yet! However, the value and importance of providing this service in an integrated and holistic fashion can not be overstated

Although new Government funding will become available in 2006, the current position is generally one of overspends in the health and social care economy, and the problem is one of 'double funding' – needing to find funding to develop a new service, whilst still having to continue funding existing services. The benefits of having 'pump-prime' funding or project funding is that it enables you to trial something you can then evaluate, and then use the outcomes to convince others to switch their funding on an 'invest to save' basis. A key 'driver for change' which influences people in health and social care, is how any service may help to achieve and maintain the 'star rating'. In the case of health and social care, achieving this will include factors like; preventing hospital admission, facilitating hospital discharge or preventing delayed discharge, assisting with waiting lists, supporting people at home and reducing admissions to residential care. It is therefore very necessary to demonstrate how assistive technology can be effective in offering solutions to these areas of concern.

Consideration also needs to be given to the use of core funding such as Access and Capacity grants, and to a creative use of alternative funding (such as E-Government grants). In the case of Local Authority Social Service Departments, as we are expected to move away from focusing on a reactive approach to those in greatest need to a more pro-active universal approach at an earlier stage, Assistive Technology fits very well with this overall prevention strategy. Think as widely as possible – make the cross-sectoral links with Community Safety and E-Government for example - and think across specialisms.

Think strategy documents

As part of the overall strategic approach, it is essential that assistive technology is positively included within key strategy documents, to have the required influence. The following are just some examples:

- Supporting People Strategy;
- Housing Strategy;
- Strategy for Older People;
- E-Government Strategy;
- Community Safety Strategy;
- Local Delivery Plans.

In the quest to convince others, it is helpful to quote from key government documents which make reference to the value of assistive technology in achieving the aims and objectives of statutory bodies (e.g. Audit Commission Report 'Keeping People Independent with Assistive Technology' 2003, Fully Equipped 2000 & 2003, NHS Plan 2000, Quality and Choice for Older peoples Housing: A strategic framework, DH ICES guidance 2001 & Telecare – Getting Started ICES 2004).

Where are we now? Next steps

Well, Norfolk is moving positively in its direction of travel. But there is still some way to go. Patience, vision and determination continue to be needed. Often it is local circumstances which provide the right climate for change, and Norfolk has just produced a number of strategic documents, which for the first time include sections on assistive technology. We have a fertile climate, the seeds of assistive technology have been sown, and we wait for them to grow.

The urban based dementia support project continues to flourish, a similar development has just begun in a rural area, we are about to commence a city based falls specific assistive technology project, and we have the beginnings of a county wide service.

The next major step is to establish a high level implementation board, and to achieve a multi-agency, countywide commitment to a joint approach to the delivery and funding of an assistive technology service across all client groups. We need to continue with and develop a major programme of awareness raising and education, which will include service users and carers, develop the opportunities for achieving an N.V.Q. in A.T., exert influence on the manufacturers and their research and development teams, look at the implications of A.T. as part of an integrated community equipment service, and the corporate issue of workforce redesign.

A further key area for development is a twenty four hour response service, available to respond to any alarms. By working in partnership and reviewing all existing out-of-hours and rapid response services, it may be possible to rationalise existing services which, with some additional input, could meet the requirements of all agencies.

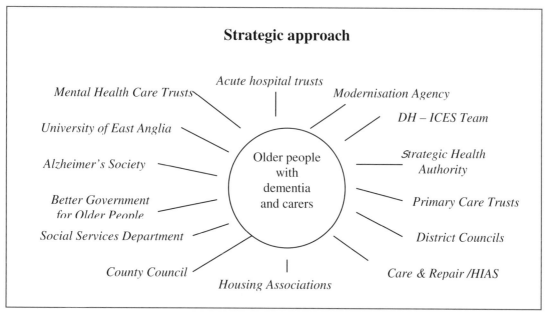

Strategic approach

Older people with dementia and carers

- Acute hospital trusts
- Mental Health Care Trusts
- University of East Anglia
- Alzheimer's Society
- Better Government for Older People
- Social Services Department
- County Council
- Housing Associations
- Modernisation Agency
- DH – ICES Team
- Strategic Health Authority
- Primary Care Trusts
- District Councils
- Care & Repair /HIAS

Some key learning points

- Partnership working is key – any assistive technology project requires a minimum of Health, SSD and Housing.
- Having the right people is essential.
- If you want to set up a project it helps to find one or two like-minded people who are entrepreneurial and have vision, energy and commitment.
- For strategic development, you need to approach different people, who are of necessity more preoccupied with performance targets and less with innovation.
- Start small - to achieve early successes.
- Establish a steering group.

- Awareness for all, education for assessors, training for key staff group.
- Recognise the anxieties and concerns of staff which technology can evoke.

- Assessment skills are key and response is crucial.
- Consider developing an intermediary, facilitative 'expert' role, which can assist busy and less knowledgeable assessment staff.
- Be aware of the importance of installation staff as partners.
- Seize any opportunity for project funding - be creative in approach.
- Engage the media, local councillors, M.P.s and 'Champions'.
- Strategic approach to funding – this needs to be multi-lateral and engage as many partners as possible.

- Be aware of other partners' drivers and performance indicators and use them.
- Ensure assistive technology is included in key strategy documents.
- Recognise the need for a high level implementation board to ensure that services are fully developed and delivered.

5. Technology in dementia care – does it bring genuine benefits?

Eileen Askham, Director of Care Services, Fold Housing Association, Northern Ireland

Introduction

Fold Housing Association was established 30 years ago to pioneer the building of traditional sheltered housing for older people. They have since diversified into general and special needs housing provision, and other care and support services. Fold are also leading providers of effective alternatives to residential care, and have become a major provider of supported housing and care services across the whole spectrum of need. Fold's Housing-with-Care schemes deliver care and support to frail older people, and two such schemes – Millbrook Court and Seven Oaks are designed to cater solely for the needs of people with dementia. This chapter will focus on the Seven Oaks scheme.

Seven Oaks

Seven Oaks in Londonderry is Fold's most recent dementia care scheme. It makes extensive use of assistive technology as a means to support people with dementia in their desire to make real, significant and sustainable improvements in their quality of life, and offer more choice and control over the services provided to them.

Built in March 2001, Seven Oaks provides housing, care and support services for:

- 14 people with mild dementia;
- 10 people with moderate dementia;
- 6 people with more severe dementia;

- There are also 5 two-bedroomed bungalows for couples, enabling them to continue living together when the dementia illness might otherwise force a separation.

In addition, 20 daily day care places provide much needed community respite in a separate purpose built day care centre.

The Alzheimer's Society operates a domiciliary care service in the community from offices based at Seven Oaks, facilitates a carers' support group, and provides an invaluable resource in respect of advice and training to Fold's residential care staff when required.

Offices for local Health & Social Services personnel, including the psycho-geriatrician, the community psychiatric nurses and the social workers of the dementia team are also provided on site, as are offices for the Getting Home & Staying Home Project. These resources are used on a daily basis.

The layout of the scheme is innovative and original. It is modelled on Londonderry city centre, and local landmarks such as the Diamond (a well-known war memorial in the centre of the city) feature as a central hub, with familiar street names leading off it. The unit is built around two internal courtyard gardens, with corridors joined by conservatory links that maximise the natural light brought into the building.

As well as individual living rooms with en suite bathrooms, there are several communal sitting rooms and dining rooms for residents to share, and a working pub which is much in demand. One street has various shops, including a grocers, a hairdresser and a chemist, all of which, with the owners' permission, are called after the same shops in the city centre. The decoration is homely and domestic and the use of old items such as manual sewing machines, gramophones, mangles, milk churns etc assist with reminiscence therapy and aid orientation.

Benefits of the scheme, as highlighted by families and carers

Evidence collected through independent evaluation and quality assurance measures suggest a range of benefits for residents.

- A person-centred, holistic care approach by staff that looks beyond the dementia illness.
- The encouragement of social interaction by staff, and the focus on helping residents to pursue personal hobbies and interests.
- The privacy afforded residents by having their own bathroom, and own personal space.
- The opportunity to make tea, do the dishes and light housework.
- The calm ambience of Seven Oaks and the fact that it is a very quiet place, with no buzzers going off or loud noise evident.
- The way in which residents are treated as individuals, and families can visit at any time.
- The approach taken to meeting the housing, care and support needs of people with dementia that improves their quality of life; as a result residents are more independent, and retain their own personal identity.
- The willingness to ensure that people with alcohol related dementia are not excluded.

Does the technology bring genuine benefits and what have been the key learning points for Fold?

Before an attempt is made to answer this question it is important to consider some of the difficulties Fold encountered in specifying, procuring, commissioning, and finally, in using assistive technology within this residential care setting for people with dementia.

As previously stated, the main objective for utilizing this new technology was a desire to make real, significant and sustainable improvements in the quality of life for individuals who are affected by dementia and to offer them more choice and control over the services provided to them.

Fold wished to determine how the technology could

- Maximise the quality of life for those suffering from dementia by providing customised care solutions.
- Maximise the efficiency and economy of the use of staff resources.
- Assist in managing risk for clients and staff.
- Enable the move from task orientation of staff to a greater relationship orientation.

Key questions that Fold were seeking to find answers to included the following:

i. *Would the use of technology reduce risk and specifically risks associated with dementia?* For example:
   Falls – people with dementia are twice as likely to fall as other older people.

Explosion – they may turn on gas hobs but forget to light them.

Fires and scalding – they may be unaware of the special dangers associated with fires, cookers, hot water etc.

Flooding – they may block the sink or toilet or leave taps running.

Wandering – they may lose track of time, confusing night with day and wander from their room in the middle of the night.

Medication- they may forget to take tablets on a regular basis.

ii. ***Would the use of technology reduce interpersonal contact?*** Would the attention of staff be diverted towards and focussed on the technology to the detriment of personal contact?

iii. ***Would the use of technology support care planning?*** Could it enable staff to be more proactive in developing individual programmes of care?

iv. ***Would the technology affect the social well-being of residents?*** Would it increase or decrease opportunities for social interaction?

v. ***Would it affect their physical well-being?*** Would residents have more control over their lives and be more independent, or would the technology increase the risk factors?

Specifying the technologies

For Fold, the deployment of technology in a residential care scheme for people with dementia was visionary and new. Knowledge of what to commission and what might be expected from the technology was limited because of the innovative nature of the scheme.

Although Fold personnel knew of the West Lothian project and the Gloucester 'Smart' house, as far as they were aware there was no other dementia care home using assistive technology in any meaningful way to support the delivery of care services, therefore there were no guidelines to follow. In addition, some elements of the technology were themselves still under development and standards of reliability unknown, so in the end, specifying what was required was approached very much on a 'try it and see' basis.

Procuring the technologies: finding suppliers

Linked to specifying were the difficulties of actually procuring the technology. There were, to begin with, a limited number of suppliers. Many of the sensors used in the scheme were literally prototypes being developed by one or two 'entrepreneurs' who believed that technology could play an increasingly important role in the delivery of care services to older people. One of the developers, operating under the name of Technology in Healthcare (TiH) was, when Fold contacted him, seeking a supplier who would undertake to turn his prototypes into products for mass production. He had been in negotiation with Tunstall Telecommunications for this purpose. Fold already operated a community alarm service using Tunstall telecommunications systems, and it seemed logical to approach Tunstall for assistance. However, until agreement between the developer and Tunstall was reached, Fold contracted directly with the developer to supply the sensors which were supported by Tunstall's baseline system.

Limited number of risk takers

Because Fold were going into unknown territory they discovered that there were few suppliers prepared to invest in producing sensors that were literally prototypes and had never been tested in situ.

Limited financial resources

The question of who should pay for the technology was also a problem. Government funding was available to build the accommodation but the technology was not accounted for in the capital costs of the scheme, therefore Fold had to consider funding the initiative themselves.

Health and Social Services did not see the technology as a 'care' cost but were very supportive of what Fold was trying to achieve and did make a small financial contribution to the overall costs.

As Supporting People was a new initiative, the Supporting People funding team were undecided as to whether the assistive technology was a care issue or a housing support matter. They would give no commitment to supporting the initiative or, indeed, the issue of technology being seen as a support service under Supporting People. At the time of writing the issue of whether Supporting People funding could be used for the deployment of technology remained unresolved.

Two years further on and with more Fold schemes under development, the same problems with procurement and finance still exist.

Commissioning the technologies

The 'lets try it and see if it works approach' presented many challenges and at times there was friction between

Fold and the suppliers due to the absence of a firm commissioning programme being in place.

Problems centred around the timescales for installing the variety of sensors and where they should be located. There was also no firm agreement about the responses required by the suppliers to deal with the malfunction of sensors; and the problems were further exacerbated by - at the time - the absence of any formal training programme for staff.

The Registration and Inspection Authority (Northern Ireland) had strong reservations about using technology to assist care delivery, were very suspicious of the technology and reluctant to see it used to its full potential. They initially insisted that only sixteen flats should be equipped with smart devices and these would be units occupied by people with the lowest levels of dependency and risk inducing behaviours. With many of the devices the greatest benefit potentially is for those people whose dementia is most severe and whose behaviour patterns most frequently give rise to risk. However, Fold have had on-going dialogue with the Registration and Inspection Authority on this issue, and the sensors are now being used throughout the scheme.

Technology provides the messages needed to enable staff to support people to remain at home or promote independence in a residential setting, but the key component to its success is the on-going customer care and support provided within the service model developed by Fold. Training provides a significant role in this respect. NVQ training ensures that customers receive a high quality service and as such NVQ level 2 was the expected level that all care staff, and staff in Fold TeleCare, (who support the development and management of the technologies), are required to attain. Fold's NVQ assessors provide advice and guidance to ensure all staff achieve this level of training. Fold's Technical Support Officer and the technology partner also provide in-house training on technology as required.

Using the technologies

Three elements of assistive technology were used at Seven Oaks.

a. Voice communication system

This first element of the assistive technology system installed allows for communication from each flat and bungalow with the Manager's office and to staff via handsets similar in appearance to mobile telephones. Residents can communicate with staff either in the main office through the speech unit on the wall or through the handsets carried by staff. Staff can also communicate with one another via the handsets. This facility provides greater freedom for the staff in carrying out their duties, e.g. they do not have to leave a resident in order to answer the telephone, if the telephone in the office is unattended. Members of staff were initially not happy about the prospect of using this technology but have subsequently recognised its value in supporting residents and are now strong advocates for its use.

b. Range of sensors

The second element of the technology system allows for a range of devices that provide alerts in pre-determined circumstances. These devices either provide information to staff about the status of a resident (that they are safely in bed or have wandered out of their room for example) or indicate that further investigation might be required.

Sensors that were used included:

A bed occupancy detector. This is set to raise an alert if a person leaves their bed and does not return within a defined period. The time delay can reflect the degree of risk attached to the resident leaving their bed without assistance. This is useful where residents may get up frequently in the night.

A furniture occupancy detector. This device performs a similar function to the bed occupancy sensor but can give reassurance to staff and relatives if absence from the bed is detected but the chair is occupied. This can be appropriate where residents with mobility problems pose no risk if seated but are in danger of having a fall if moving about unsupervised. Members of staff are trained to respond by exploring any underlying reasons for the sensors to activate – this helps to ensure that the technology is used to support rather than control the behaviour of residents.

Automatic light controls. These permit lights to come on automatically when movement is detected. For example a resident getting up in the night to go to the toilet triggers lighting in the bedroom and in the toilet. The intensity of light can be adjusted to aid orientation: thus the light in the toilet is stronger to provide direction to the toilet, which is usually where the resident needs to go when they get up in the night.

A door opening detector. This raises an alert if a door is opened either by someone entering or by someone leaving. Thus a resident going out of their room in the night will raise an alert and prompt investigation by staff. Alternatively if another person enters the room, perhaps another resident who is disoriented and wandering, staff will be prompted to investigate. These devices can be fitted to the entrance doors of all flats occupied by residents who may be prone to wander.

A fall detector – this is fitted to the clothing of the resident and will detect a fall, triggering an alert to summon assistance.

An incontinence alert – this device can be used with incontinence pads and will detect a level of saturation before the capacity of the pad has been reached. This allows a timely intervention before bedclothes are wet. Alternatively it may allow a resident who might otherwise be woken to check their state of continence to sleep on undisturbed. However, there are difficulties with current models of this device in comfort in use and acceptability to users and care staff. At the time of writing Fold decided not to continue to use this device until acceptable changes to the design of the technology have been made.

A flood detector. This raises an alert and turns off the water supply if flooding is detected in the kitchen or bathroom.

An excess heat detector. If residents have access to kitchen areas this raises an alert and turns off the power if oven or hob is left on.

Environmental controls. The bungalows are equipped with additional devices that control the fridge, microwave, kettles etc and are designed to offer extra support to the couples who live there.

c. MIDAS System (otherwise known as the 'Modular Intelligent Domiciliary Alarm System')

The third element in the system is the Super Midas system: a computer that receives data from the devices located in residents' rooms and provides graphic representation of the status of the resident. MIDAS also provides a historical record of all alarms triggered by the sensors and thereby contributes to the person-centred care planning process.

Using the technologies and approach to resolution of problems

Gaining the acceptance of staff to the new technology, and their commitment to making it work was the biggest hurdle Fold had to overcome. To do this, Fold management adopted an open attitude toward the difficulties that were being encountered, welcoming suggestions from staff and a willingness to make changes to improve the situation. They continued to press the suppliers to rectify faults and to provide support to staff in commissioning the equipment. The appointment of a manager whose responsibilities included the operation of the Seven Oaks site in general and the implementation of the technology in particular greatly improved the situation.

A suggestion that two 'champions' be appointed from within the staff to provide peer support to staff and reinforcement of training on a day-to-day basis was made by technology suppliers. The suggestion was taken up and has proved highly successful. These two champions also took on the basic maintenance of the system: re-setting devices, reporting faults, and so on. The role has also proved to be a useful vehicle for staff development.

Initiatives were taken locally to strengthen practice in the use of all the technologies. A protocol was drafted and an instruction leaflet for care staff produced, using information from suppliers' literature in a user-friendly format.

Now that the initial problems with the technology have been largely resolved, it is evident that further evaluation of the sensors will be needed before all the benefits in care practice can be substantiated.

Have the key questions raised when consideration was given to using assistive technology been answered?

i. *Have Fold been able to reduce risk?*
    In some cases risk has been reduced, for example, the risk of flooding, but it would perhaps be more appropriate to say that risks are more effectively managed. For example, the door sensors enabled staff to manage more appropriately a resident who was prone to leave his room during the night, enter another room and begin to stack up furniture, creating a risk for both himself and the other person. Staff could respond and intervene immediately an alert was triggered, thus preventing this situation from arising.

ii. *Has interpersonal contact decreased as a result of using technology?*
    Staff have been able to dedicate *more* time on a one-to-one basis to residents. Previously, the only way of knowing that a resident was safe and well during the night was to carry out hourly checks. Sensors mean that staff are not driven by 'hourly' routines, and can dedicate more personal time to residents who may be restless, or unable to sleep during the night.

iii. *Is care planning better informed?*
    Technology has enable staff to be proactive in practice instead of reactive. The information provided by the technology identifies emerging patterns and trends in a resident's physical abilities. It helps identify increasing mobility or dexterity problems, for example. As a result care planning is better informed on issues such mobility, etc and staff can seek professional help and advice at a much earlier stage.

iv. *Has there been any difference in the social well-being of residents?*
    The need for staff to constantly monitor and supervise residents is greatly reduced because staff have the confidence to know that alerts will be triggered by the sensors should a resident be in any difficulty. This enables staff to focus much more time and attention on social activities and social interaction with the residents, helping to keep residents active and engaged with life.

v. *Has there been any improvement in the physical well-being of residents?*
    Fold's experience is that technology has also contributed to improvements in physical well-being. For example, fall detectors alert staff immediately a resident has a fall. The result is that medical assistance can be sought, if required, more quickly. Families are also reassured that their loved one is not lying somewhere unattended, because members of staff do not know a fall has occurred. Bedroom and bathroom lights automatically coming on when a person gets out of bed at night reduces the risk of falls occurring. The reduction of this kind of risk results in improved physical well-being. Using technology has also resulted in medication of a sedative nature being reduced for residents. As a result, their quality of life has been greatly enhanced, since they are more alert and mobile during the day.

Benefits of using assistive technology

Fold have identified ten principle benefits from using technology at the present time.

i. It supports the development of less intrusive practice. Residents do not need to be checked routinely to see that they are in their bed, are not lying on the floor, are not in a cold environment at risk of hypothermia, or that their continence pad is about to be overwhelmed.

ii. Risk to residents can be reduced. Sensors will raise an alert either at once, or after an appropriate interval, therefore detection does not rely on the next hourly check that may be 59 minutes away. A response can be made at once, reducing risk and improving the prospects for recovery, as in the case of a stroke or a fall resulting in a fracture for example.

iii. Some situations of risk can be pre-empted. By observing changes in behaviour pattern detected by the system, staff may be able to predict adverse incidents, such as a fall. Upgrading of software at Seven Oaks is planned to further strengthen that capability.

iv. Staff can work more confidently. A situation in which residents need their attention or are at risk is automatically brought to their notice through the operation of the system. The ability of staff to communicate with one another without leaving residents allows a higher level of mutual support and access to assistance when required.

v. Staff can focus on quality interventions. The release of time from routine visual checks allows time to be spent on quality interventions with residents. In addition to the therapeutic gain for residents, this enriches the experience of staff, contributing to a better quality of care.

vi. The information recorded by the MIDAS system provides *informs care planning* and supports the person-centred approach to the delivery of care.

vii. It reassures relatives. For example, when a daughter approached the Manager deeply concerned by the fact that her mother was telling her that she had fallen in the night and had been lying on the floor for an hour before anyone attended to her, the Manager was able to produce a print-out generated by the technology which proved that staff had actually responded within one minute of the alarm being raised by the fall detector. This greatly reassured the daughter.

viii. It challenges assumptions made about people with dementia – for example, that people with dementia cannot be trusted to have a kettle in their room, a cooker in their flat, or a plug in their wash hand basin. Some of the technologies can assist personal mobility and functionality for people with dementia.

ix. It supports the delivery of quality services. Residents have greater choice and control over their lives. One of the male residents had been a chef before he retired. Every Saturday morning he prepares a cooked breakfast for himself and three other male residents, and they share it together in one of the small dining rooms. The technology supports staff in their desire to assist residents in maintaining those daily living skills that encourage independence.

x. It drives creativity and innovation. Staff using the technology have provided invaluable information to the developers about the capacity of the technology in use and have challenged them to seek to improve or expand the range of sensors available, such as the need to change the size and shape of the incontinence sensors to make them more acceptable to the user.

Key learning points

The following are the key learning points that have emerged from Fold Housing Associations use of technology in residential care settings.

- The specification of the technology must set out in general terms the outcomes expected, allowing the suppliers to respond with a technical schedule.
- The configuration of devices should reflect the needs of residents rather than adopting an 'all available devices in every location'.
- Registration and Inspection authorities and other key stakeholders need to be fully briefed and 'signed up' to the purpose of the technology and involved in commissioning, monitoring and induction.
- Adequate arrangements for, and investment in, staff training need to be in place if the system is to operate successfully and the confidence of staff is to be strengthened.
- A champion or champions drawn from the staff be identified to resolve minor problems and, through peer support, encourage the use of the technology. They can explain how the system operates, and the information it provides, in plain language to staff, residents and relatives.

- There needs to be a clear statement of care philosophy and objectives in place to guide the specification of the technology.

And finally,

- it is vital that the care philosophy drives technology, and that the technology does not drive the care philosophy.

Conclusion

Whilst Seven Oaks remains a 'flagship' location for Fold, supporting their drive for innovation, it is true to say that a number of the elements of the original technology infrastructure are now in a position to be upgraded.

Within the last two years, and since Seven Oaks was opened, some new approaches to the implementation of supporting technology have been developed to a prototype stage by Tunstall Telecommunications.

Fold is committed to implementing some of these new items alongside the existing infrastructure in order to ensure that Seven Oaks continues to fulfil its visionary role, and that the momentum generated by Seven Oaks in using assistive technology to support care delivery for people with dementia is maintained and enhanced.

References

Appleton, N., & Shreeve, M., (2004) *New Technology and the Housing-with-Care Scheme for People with Dementia at Seven Oaks. Londonderry.* (Contract Consulting Old Chapel Publishing Bell Lane Cassington Oxfordshire OX29 4DS).

6. Reflections on ethics, dementia and technology

Clive Baldwin, Senior Lecturer, Bradford Dementia Group, University of Bradford

Introduction

It is not surprising that there has been a marked increase in interest in using and developing technology in dementia care. The failing capacities of individuals would seem to lend themselves to a technological solution, be that solution devices to use in the home, Smart Houses, electronic tagging or ubiquitous computing. Technology, however, is not without its cost, not only in financial terms, but also in terms of our relationships, our physical environment and our sense of self but also our ethical thinking and environment.

In this chapter I am less interested in discussing specific applications of technology but rather some of the underlying philosophical and ethical issues regarding technology *per se* and its application in the field of dementia care. In so doing I hope to draw attention to ethical matters that do not yet seem to have found a place in the literature on technology, ethics and dementia. Before doing so, however, it is important to note that this chapter is not a review of the literature, nor do I claim that it is comprehensive in its coverage. My aims are far more humble.

Furthermore, some of the issues raised may seem to conflict with each other. That is as it should be, for I am not attempting to produce a cohesive ethics of technology in dementia care but simply to draw attention and generate debate. It must also be remembered that there is, and always will be, conflict (or at least disagreement) when ethical issues are discussed. The four principles of bioethics - autonomy, beneficence, non-malfeasance and justice - for example, do not always sit comfortably together (see Beauchamp and Childress 2001).

Definitions and scope

Definitions of technology may be narrower or more encompassing according to the purposes of the discussion. At one end of the spectrum the term might be used as a synonym for tool or machine, at the other it can be seen as "the application of organized knowledge to practical tasks by ordered systems of people and machines" (Barbour 1992: 3). The latter definition has the advantage of allowing for different *technologies* and is comprehensive enough to encompass the four major types of technologies identified by Martin *et al* (1988): the technologies of production, which permit us to produce, transform, or manipulate things; the technologies of sign systems, which permit us to use signs, meanings, symbols, or signification; the technologies of power, which determine the conduct of individuals and submit them to certain ends or domination; and technologies of the self, which permit individuals to effect by their own means or with the help of others a certain number of operations on their own bodies and souls, thoughts, conduct, and way of being. In this way of viewing things, discussion of technologies would include discussion of assessment tools such as the Mini-Mental State Examination (MMSE) or the Dementia Care Mapping tool. This, however, is too ambitious a project for this paper and consequently I will limit my reflections to the ethical issues arising from the development and application of physical technology. In particular I will draw illustrations from three broad areas: tools such as automatic shut off devices, electronic tags, alarms and calendars (see for example, Penhale & Manthorpe 2001, Woolham & Frisby 2002, the Tunstall Group 2003 and Miskelly 2004); Information and Communications Technology such as telephone support lines, tele-medicine and carers' support lists (see, for example, Colantonio et. al. 2001 and Czaja & Rubert 2002); and developments in providing a technological environment, such as Smart Houses (see, for example, Bjørneby 2000 and Chapman 2001) and ubiquitous computing (see, for example, Mihailidis & Fernie 2002, Morris & Lundell 2003 and Rice 2003).

Philosophy and technology

Although there has been considerable interest shown in the development of technology (ASTRID 2000, Bjørneby *et al* 1999, Morris & Lundell 2003) there is little in the literature that addresses questions raised by the philosophy of technology. In developing technology for use in dementia care, there has been some debate on the ethical issues involved (see below) but not on the wider issues of what affect technology has on our ways of perceiving and being in the world. The relationship between technology and society is complex and dynamic and while we may influence and channel technological development according to our values, aims and desires, technology also impacts *upon* those values, aims and desires. Skolimowski (1983), for example, points out that thinking technologically is to think in terms of accuracy, durability and efficiency. This is clearly illustrated in Wendell Berry's refusal to write using a computer. Berry (1997) reports that

although a computer would enable him to write faster, his concern is to write *better,* a quality that the computer cannot help him in developing.

Other writers, such as Jarvie (1983) and Mitcham (1994), comment on technology and the structure of knowledge. We live in a technology-saturated world and how we think about technology and the relationship between technology and society is partly determined, or at least heavily influenced by that technological environment (see Araya 1995 for a discussion of this with regard to ubiquitous computing). The danger here is that if we do not reflect upon the nature of that environment we are more likely to be influenced subconsciously by it. So, in the case of dementia care, we may want to reflect upon whether accuracy, durability and efficiency are or paramount importance when thinking about using and developing technology.

A second strand of philosophical reflection concerning technology is raised by Cooper (1995) when he discusses the impact of technology and technological thinking on the person. Citing Roszak (1983), Cooper argues that because technology promotes some human capacities over others, what it is to be a person comes to be defined in terms of those capacities – for example, the narrowing of knowledge to the acquisition and processing of information. In part, this 'technologising' of the self can help explain the hyper-cognitive society that Post identifies as devaluing people with dementia (Post 1995). In promoting one particular view of what it is to be human, technology can push other views and other aspects of being human to the sidelines:

'Within a society geared to technological progress, and honouring the faculties which contribute to it, moral conviction, religious sense, taste and sensibility play only bit parts. They are then relegated to the realm of the merely 'subjective'... The implication, of course, is that taste, morality and religion do not constitute a person's being: they belong, rather, on the smorgasbord from which the person – essentially a creature of knowledge and reason, but regrettably unable to live by these alone – can pick and choose at will'

Cooper (1995: p. 17).

The concept of the self is a subject of great debate within the field of dementia (see, for example, Herskowits 1995, Post 1995, Hughes 2001) yet there is little, if anything, in the literature addressing the impact of technology on people with dementia or their carers. Such discussions as there are may mention such things as the need to design technology that is not deficit-focused in order to preserve the self-esteem of the person with dementia, but there is, as yet, nothing on how the person with dementia is redefined or reconstructed in his or her relationship to technology. For example, to what extent is the Self reconstituted through living with ubiquitous computing where technology is attributed "the right to drive by itself the way in which certain aspects of everyday life are lived", a way of thinking that "exhibits a highly unreflective submission to the powers of technology" (Araya 1995: p.236).

A third strand in the philosophy of technology that has implications for dementia care is the impact of technology on our form of life or life

as a whole. Cooper (1995) makes two points in relation to this. First, the rate of technological change impairs the capacity to see life as a whole, that is, seeing life as having a predictable shape and structure; and, second, that technology erodes intimate human relationships. With regard to dementia care, these potential dangers perhaps need even more attention. The onset and progression of dementia has devastating impacts upon one's capacities to engage in the world. Forgetfulness may fragment the shape and structure of one's world and the introduction of technology, however well-intended, may exacerbate the problem. On the other hand, technology may be designed to restore or enhance one's sense of predictability and structure. For example, it is possible to maintain a sense of one's life through reminiscence therapy and there have been attempts to develop technology that enables people's reminiscences (Gowans et. al. 2004).

There are two aspects to the danger of the erosion of intimate human relationships. The first – perhaps the most discussed although probably the less dangerous – is the reduction of human contact through the safety and surveillance provided by the application of technological solutions. If, the reasoning goes, the person is safe and can be monitored via a range of technological devices, then there is less reason for her or him to be checked on in person. The lessened opportunities for human contact are seen as resulting in further isolation on the part of the person with dementia. This argument, however, may romanticise the quality of the contact between people with dementia and others. Social care services, under pressure of resource scarcity and budget restraints often allow a minimum of time for service provision and contact is task oriented (the provision of meals, cleaning, bathing and so on). Furthermore, often such tasks are the responsibility of different people, and so people with dementia may be faced with a constant stream of people with whom they have no significantly meaningful relationship. Participants in my own research quite often reported that their relative required companionship more than service. If this is the case, then technology should be aimed at easing the task so that more time can be spent in simply being with the person with dementia. On an anecdotal level, one carer participating in the ENABLE research (described later in this chapter) and evaluating the item locator reported that the device reduced the time she spent looking for her mother's belongings thus increasing the time she could spend with her mother without such distractions.

The second danger of the erosion of human intimacy is one that, as far as I am aware, has never been addressed in the literature on technology and dementia - that the nature of the contact between the person with dementia and the carer will become technologically determined. In other words, what human contact there is will focus on and be mediated by technology. The question here is, does a technological solution move the relationship away from person cared for/person caring towards user of technology/technology support worker? Technology is deeply insinuated into people's perceptions, thoughts and behaviours yet there is no discussion of the impact of dementia care technology on these. The concern here is that the I-Thou relationship is displaced by an I-It-Thou relationship. This displacement may take two forms.

First, interactions between the carer-technician and the person with dementia focus on the technology – for example, in the exchange, "How are you getting on with the automated pill dispenser? Is it working properly? Can I see if it is set correctly?" and so on. Second, the person with dementia becomes known through the technology: for example, equipment that monitors patterns of behaviour may produce a picture of opening and shutting doors that appears erratic and thus the person is typified as someone who erratically opens and shuts doors. The monitoring equipment cannot identify meaning and purpose behind such behaviours. In both these examples, the technology has mediated the direct relationship between the person with dementia and the carer.

Values and technology

Technology is not, as some would claim and as is widely assumed, value neutral and that value judgments only enter into the debate when discussing the application of technology. Far from it:

> 'The values and world views, the intelligence and stupidity, the biases and vested interests of those who design, accept and maintain a technology are embedded in the technology itself'

> Staudenmaier (1985: p. 165).

This is easily demonstrated: electronic tagging devices reflect the value placed on surveillance regardless of to whom they are applied, guns reflect the value placed on the capacity to kill regardless of the circumstances in which they are employed and Smart Houses reflect the value placed on autonomy and safety regardless of how they are used.

There is no one best way to design a technology – different stakeholders may have different perceptions of what is needed, how it is to be realised and what the criteria for success might be. The design that finally emerges as the 'best' will be the one that best reflects the values and interests of those involved in that design. For example, there was nothing logical or necessary about the final design of the bicycle, the development of which involved diverse technical specifications, aimed at diverse users with diverse criteria for success (Barbour 1992).

For Marcuse (1964) domination was built into technology through the technological rationality that underlay the technology and what was required was to develop a new rationality in which technology was reconstructed around a notion of the good, which for Marcuse was fundamentally concerned with realizing inherent potentialities:

> *'Consequently, what is at stake is the redefinition of values in technical terms, as elements in the technological process. The new ends, as technical ends, would then operate in the project and in the construction of the machinery, and not only in its utilization'*

> Marcuse, (1964: p. 232).

Technological design for dementia is no different – the question is, however, what are the values that we want to build into that technology? This, in essence, is an ethical question and our answer will determine our ethical stance.

It is here that the principles of 'Design for All' would seem to be highly relevant for technological development in dementia care. The seven principles of 'Design for All' are intended to guide the design process so that products and environments are inclusive and accessible. These principles are:

Equitable use. The design is useful and marketable to people with diverse abilities. This has the advantage that design does not stigmatise people with dementia by either focusing on their cognitive or functional deficits or by requiring a level of ability over and above those of which they are capable.

Flexibility in use. The design should accommodate a wide range of individual preferences and abilities including the provision of choice in the methods of use and an adaptability to the user's pace. This is particularly important with regard to people with dementia as choice can engender a sense of control and autonomy and adaptability to pace does not set up the person to fail in using the technology.

Simple and intuitive use. The use of the design should be easy to understand, regardless of the user's experience, knowledge, language skills, or current concentration level.

Perceptible information. The design should communicate necessary information effectively to the user, regardless of ambient conditions or the user's sensory abilities, that is, use different modes of presentation (such as pictorial, verbal and tactile), maximise the legibility of essential information and eliminate redundant information. This principle would help eliminate confusing extraneous information and allow for use of the product by those with varying degrees of dementia.

Tolerance for error. The design should minimise hazards and the adverse consequences of accidental or unintended actions.

Low physical effort. The design should be able to be used efficiently and comfortably and with a minimum of fatigue.

Size and space for approach and use. Appropriate size and space should be provided for approach, reach, manipulation, and use regardless of user's body size, posture, or mobility.

(see http://www.design.ncsu.edu/cud/univ_design/princ_overview.htm).

A recent research project – ENABLE – funded by the European Commission under the programme 'Quality of Life and Management of Living Resources' tested and evaluated a number of technological products for use with people with dementia including technical devices to support memory, facilitate communication and provide pleasure and activity. (see www.enableproject.org). Items were selected or designed for the project on the basis of the above principles. The ENABLE project developed and evaluated the following products:

- Day-night calendar aimed at orienting the person with dementia;
- An item locator that set of an auditory signal from a tab fixed to commonly misplaced items such as keys, purse, handbag and so on;
- A cooker usage monitor that will switch off the gas if a pan is over-heating;
- A medication dispenser with auditory signal to remind the person with dementia that it was time to take her or his medication;
- A picture gramophone that allows people with dementia to select

familiar tunes through touch-screen technology;
- Bath water level and temperature monitor and controller;
- Remote day planner aimed at a close relative or carer being able to write the actual day's appointments or happenings via the Internet, to aid the memory of the user with dementia;
- Programmable telephone with large buttons. Photos of persons frequently called can be put on the buttons for one touch dialling.
- An automatic bedroom light that switches on should the person get out of bed;

While the numbers or participants involved in the evaluation of the use and usefulness of the products was somewhat small, the ENABLE project has gone some way to raising an awareness of the potential of technology to enhance the quality of dementia care and clearly indicates that values can be consciously embedded into the design and application of technological devices.

Ethics, ethical frameworks and dementia

Ethics, too, is about values, whether these values stem from a sense of what it means to be a person, our sense of duties or rights or our relationships (to ourselves, each other and the world). The reasons we hold to such values - tradition, religion, philosophical reflection, family loyalty or simply habit - are outwith the purview of this chapter. It is important, however, to note that the values we stand by and our reasons for doing so are multiple and varied. In ethical theory as well as in everyday life there are competing views as to what are (and what should be) our values and what constitute good foundations for those values.

Over the last five years there have been a number of reports focusing on the ethics of the use and development of technology in dementia care (ASTRID 2000, Bjørneby et. al. 1999). For the authors of these reports the main challenges confronting the use of technology in dementia care have been those posed by challenging behaviour, and much technology has been geared towards the surveillance and control of people who 'wander' or other safety issues. While other applications of technology are acknowledged – such as assistance in the planning and co-ordination of care or providing memory aids or stimulus for people with dementia until recently these have been the subject of less attention. The ENABLE project mentioned above has gone some way to addressing the under-explored potential of technology.

Whatever the aim of the technology, however, most of the discussion in the literature on ethics, technology and dementia focuses on how technology may impinge, enhance or fit with the bio-ethical principles (see Downs 1997, Bjørneby et. al. 1999) of autonomy, beneficence, non-maleficence and justice. In this, the literature is probably simply reflecting the dominance of the bio-ethical principle-ist approach in health care generally, but might also be explained in part by the nature of the technology already being developed: the links between surveillance technology and civil liberties, and technology designed to protect the person with dementia and beneficence being obvious. It must be remembered, however, that the bio-ethical principle-ist framework, while providing some guidance in the application of technology, is not the only ethical framework that can be drawn upon in discussing technology and dementia. Other frameworks, such

as the ethics of care (see Noddings 1984), might prompt us to ask different questions of technology. For example, while bio-ethical discussion tends to focus on the individual the ethics of care focuses more on relationships and communication. A principle-ist approach to a particular item of technology might then ask the question, 'Does this technology enhance the autonomy of the individual?' An alternative approach – that of the ethics of care – might ask, 'Does this technology bring people together in interdependence?' or, 'Does this technology enhance the focal practice of caring? (Michelfelder, 2004).

One example of a technological innovation that can be seen as potentially enhancing inter-dependence is the development of help and support lines for carers of people with dementia. One such project was reported at a recent international conference, (ENABLE, Oslo, Norway June 2004) This project, under the auspices of Vestfold University College, Norway involves providing a system and the technology for carers to be able to support each other (and seek specialized nursing advice) via video-phone link and to access information regarding dementia via an intranet. This project is, at the time of writing, in its early stages but its potential for bringing people together in mutually supportive ways is clear.

The ethical framework we use to evaluate and analyse technology will determine the sorts of questions that can be asked of that technology and the boundaries within which ethical reflection can legitimately take place. Much work is required to explore the differing landscapes carved out by bioethics, feminist ethics, narrative ethics and virtue ethics, to name but a few of the potential frameworks for ethical analysis.

Ethics and technology

Ethics and technology relate to each other in complex and dynamic ways. It is not a case of simply applying ethical standards upon the design and application of technology (although this, of course is vital) but also reflecting upon how the technological environment we live in impacts upon the nature of ethical reflection itself. Jonas (2004) argues that the development of technology has rendered the presumptions of traditional ethical theories obsolete and that human nature has changed with the development of technology. For writers such as Illich, ethics is impossible under a regime of scarcity where ethical action is determined by utility (1996). Others, such as Jacques Ellul, argue that rather than negating ethics

> 'The power and autonomy of technique are so well secured that it, in turn, has become the judge of what is moral, the creator of a new morality'

> Ellul, (1964: p.134).

Each of these views poses a challenge to those who argue that ethics applies only to the design and application of technology – for each of these raise questions as to the structure and scope of ethical action.

In a technological society moral action is that which is permitted or determined by the requirements of technology. For example, what is technologically possible may become morally acceptable or desirable: be it stem cell research, cloning, genetic modification of crops or the development of ubiquitous computing.

In order to properly assess the role that technology has to play in dementia care we need, somehow, to be able to step back and understand how technology has helped to frame the ethical questions as well as how it might be ethically applied as a solution. This ethical reflection is no mere distraction or a luxury that can await less pressing times. Without clarity and agreement on what the ethical questions to be addressed by technology are, we run the risk of having those questions posed for us by the autonomous development of technology (see Ellul 1964). Ethics, in these circumstances becomes reactive rather than proactive.

Unintended consequences

With any solution to any problem, and with any application of technology, there is the possibility of unintended consequences (Winner 2004). Merton (1976) identified potential sources of unintended consequences including ignorance, error and the 'imperious immediacy of interest', that is, people want the intended consequences so much that they choose to ignore any unintended effect.

Two examples will suffice to illustrate this: the first, the case of automatic doors; the second, central heating. The usefulness and desirability of these inventions is unquestioned. Both, however, have had unintended consequences. Automatic doors, for instance, while providing access to all, have also removed the opportunity to hold open doors for people and thus lessened the opportunity for making convivial contact (however brief) with other human beings. The human interaction of 'please', 'thank you', 'may I help you?', 'after you', the smiles, the eye contact and the feelings of having helped basically all disappear in the presence of automatic doors. I have no doubt that the intentions behind the development of automatic doors were benevolent and the benefit of the technology is not in dispute - but benevolence and benefit come at a cost and we need to be aware of such costs if we are to make informed decisions as to the design and application of any given technology.

While automatic doors displace human contact, central heating replaces both meaning and meaningful activity. The stove, which central heating replaces, was more than just a means of heating a room, it was

> '...a focus, a hearth, a place that gathered the work and leisure of a family and gave the house a center. Its coldness marked the morning, and the spreading of its warmth the beginning of the day. It assigned to the different family members tasks that defined their place in the household. The mother built the fire, the children kept the firebox filled, and the father cut the firewood. It provided for the entire family a regular and bodily engagement with the rhythm of the seasons that was woven together of the threat of cold and the solace of warmth, the smell of wood smoke, the exertion of sawing and of carrying, the teaching of skills, and the fidelity to daily tasks.'

> Borgmann, (2004: p. 116).

One would be hard pushed to argue that, even with its considerable advantages, central heating embodies or represents anything like the stove. In terms of the design and application of technology we should take into account those focal things and practices that will be positively or adversely affected by the technology.

Technological development can, of course, reduce the burden of caring. Help-lines and video-phones can provide personal (if not geographically proximate) contact and support; automatic shut-off devices may provide safety and electronic tags may alleviate carer anxiety where people with dementia may go for a walk and get lost. What these devices cannot do, however, is provide a sense of place or meaning in the care-giving relationship. The danger inherent with the development of technology is that sense of place and meaning is displaced by a technological solution to a technologically determined problem. To be truly person-centred technology in dementia care needs to give priority to the roles, relationships and meanings experienced by people with dementia and their carers in their own, unique situations.

While it is impossible to foresee everything that might happen as a result of developing technology (however well-designed and however well it embeds the values that we have deliberately designed into it) it is important to think about such potential consequences and, if possible, address these at the design stage. One way of doing this may be to include the widest range of people in the design of such technology. Bringing together different perspectives, especially those of the end-users of technology whose focal concerns and practices will ultimately be affected, may go some way to forestalling some of the unintended consequences of developing technology for use in dementia care. In this way, different priorities and foci may be built into the technology and thus prevent the loss of contact, meaning and meaningful activity.

Concluding remarks

In conclusion I want to make a number of suggestions regarding how we might approach the question of technological development in dementia care. This is by no means a comprehensive programme, merely some indications of the things that we should perhaps think about along the way.

The first, and perhaps most obvious, question is whether the situation calls for a technological solution. The problem of 'wandering', for example, does not necessarily call for greater technological surveillance but could be addressed through the availability of walking companions. In my own research into the ethical issues for family carers of people with dementia one carer was very clear that wandering was not a problem because he simply went with his wife wherever she wanted to go. This forestalled any conflict between the couple because the wife did not feel constrained by her husband and it also maintained the continuity of their relationship in which they had always done things together. Of course, this may not be a practical solution in every case but the point is well made – that human rather than technological solutions may be more beneficial or appropriate. In thinking about the application of technology, therefore, it may be worth thinking first about whether the problem can be addressed in non-technological ways.

The second general point I want to make is that perhaps the ethical issues involved in the use and development of technology in dementia care are only different in degree rather than nature from the ethical issues that are raised for us all by advancing technology. Technology designed for safety, control and surveillance surrounds us all – from seat-belts and airbags to car tracking devices and the worst excesses of the intelligence services. We also make use of a far greater range of technology than previous generations and adapt ourselves to it more or less willingly – for example, the now near necessity to be computer literate if one is to find employment.

One concern with regard to technology and dementia is that the person with dementia will not be in control of, nor understand the workings of the technology being used. This concern is, of course, real, but in this people with dementia are not really any different from the rest of us. Much of the technology that surrounds us is not of our making, is beyond our understanding and is in the control of others - from CCTVs in the car park to the financial monitoring systems of credit houses, from air traffic control to identity cards. Who we are, how we relate and what values we wish to embed in our technology are questions for us all, not just for those working in dementia care. As such those involved in dementia care should seriously engage with the philosophy of technology.

A third point is that the use and development of technology is morally ambiguous. Even when ethical values are consciously embedded within the design of a technological device, there is always a cost involved, something is lost or displaced. Of course, the benefits gained by deploying the technology may far outweigh the losses – but these losses, be they social and/or psychological, should form part of the equation in evaluating technology.

Finally, and perhaps most importantly, we need a more proactive ethics. Rather than responding to developments we would, perhaps, be better to work out and agree in advance what sort of values and ethical considerations we want technology to adhere to. In this the ENABLE project has made headway but there is still much to be done. We should not limit ourselves to the ethical questions raised by the principle-ist approach to ethics but look to other ethical frameworks for guidance and evaluation. Ultimately our considerations about technology and dementia are about care and relationships; perhaps caring and interdependence should be at the heart of our ethical considerations.

References

Araya, A.A., (1995) Questioning ubiquitous computing. *Proceedings of the 1995 ACM 23rd Annual Conference on Computer Science.* New York: ACM Press. Available from: http://portal.acm.org/citation.cfm?id=259560&dl=ACM&coll=portal (Accessed February 2005).

Barbour, I., (1992) Ethics in an age of technology. London: SCM Press.

Beauchamp, T., & Childress, J., (2001) The principles of bioethics. New York: Oxford University Press.

Berry, W., (1997) *Why I won't buy a computer.* Available from: http://www.tipiglen.dircon.co.uk/berry not.html (Accessed February 2005).

Bjørneby, S., (2000) *Smart Houses: can they Really Benefit Older People?* Signpost, 5 (2): 36-38.

Bjørneby, S., Topo, P., & Holthe, T., (1999) Technology, Ethics and Dementia: A guidebook on how to apply technology in dementia care

INFO-banken: Norwegian Centre for Dementia Research.

Borgmann, A., (2004) *Focal Things and Practices.* In, Kaplan, D.M., (ed) Readings in the philosophy of technology. Lanham: Rowman and Littlefield Publishers.

Chapman, A., (2001) *There's no Place like a Smart Home.* Journal of Dementia Care, 9 (1): 28-31.

Colantonio, A., Cohen, C., & Pon, M., (2001) *Assessing Support Needs of Caregivers of Persons with Dementia: Who wants what?* Community Mental Health Journal, 37 (3): 231-243.

Cooper, D.E., (1995) *Technology: Liberation or Enslavement?* In Fellows, R. (ed)., Philosophy and technology. Cambridge: Cambridge University Press.

Czaja, S.J. & Rubert, M.P., (2002) *Telecommunications Technology as an Aid to Family Caregivers of Persons with Dementia.* Psychosomatic Medicine, 64 (3): 469-476.

Downs, M., (1997) *Assessing ethical issues in the use of technology for people with dementia.* In, Bjørneby, S., & Van Berlo, A., (eds.) Ethical Issues in the Use of Technology in Dementia Care. Knegsel: Akontes Publishing.

Ellul, J., (1964) The Technological Society. New York: Knopf.

Gowans, G., Campbell, J., Alm, N., Dye, R., Astell, A. & Ellis, M., (2004) *Designing a multimedia conversation aid for reminiscence therapy in dementia care environments.* Conference on Human Factors in Computing Systems Extended abstracts: 825 – 836. Available from:

http://portal.acm.org (Accessed February 2005).

Herskovits, E., (1995) *Struggling over Subjectivity: Debates about the "Self" and Alzheimer's Disease.*, Medical Anthropology Quarterly 9 (2, June): 146-164.

Hughes J.C., (2001) *Views of the Person with Dementia.* Journal of Medical Ethics, 27 (2nd April): 86-91.

Illich, I., (1996) *The Wisdom of Leopold Kohr.* Resurgence, 184. Available from: http://homepage.mac.com/tinapple/illich/1996_illich_kohr.html (Accessed February 2005).

Jarvie, I.C., (1983) *Technology and the Structure of Knowledge.* In Mitcham, C. and Mackey, R. (eds). Philosophy and Technology: Readings in the philosophical problems of technology. New York: The Free Press.

Jonas, H., (2004) *Technology and Responsibility.* In Kaplan, D.M., (ed.) Readings in the Philosophy of Technology. Lanham: Rowman and Littlefield Publishers.

Marcuse, H., (1964) One-dimensional Man: Studies in the ideology of advanced industrial society. Available from: http://cartoon.iguw.tuwien.ac.at/christian/marcuse/odm9.html (Accessed February 2005).

Martin, L.H., Gutman, H., & Hutton, P.H., (1988) *Technologies of the Self: A Seminar with Michel Foucault.* London: Tavistock., pp.16-49.

Marshall, M., (ed.) (2000) ASTRID: A social and technological response to meeting the needs of individuals with dementia and their carers. London: Hawker.

Merton, R.K., (1976) *The Unanticipated Consequences of Purposive Social Action.* In Merton, R.K., Sociological Ambivalence and Other Essays. New York: Free Press.

Michelfelder, D.P., (2004) *Technological Ethics in a Different Voice.* In Kaplan, D.M., (ed.) Readings in the Philosophy of Technology. Lanham: Rowman and Littlefield Publishers.

Mihailidis, A., & Fernie, G., (2002) *Context aware assistive devices for older adults with dementia.* Gerontechnology, 2 (2): 173-189.

Miskelly, F., (2004) *A novel system of electronic tagging in patients with dementia and wandering.* Age and Ageing, 33 (3): 304-306

Mitcham, C., (1994) Thinking Through Technology: The path between engineering and philosophy. Chicago: University of Chicago Press.

Morris, M., & Lundell, J., (2003) *Ubiquitous Computing for Cognitive Decline: Findings from Intel's Proactive Health Research. Intel Corporation.* Available from: http://www.alz.org/Research/Care/Intel_UbiquitousComputing.pdf (Accessed February 2005).

Noddings, N., (1984) Caring: A Feminine Approach to Ethics and Moral Education. Berkeley: University of California Press.

Penhale, B., & Manthorpe, J., (2001) *Using Electronic Aids to Assist People with Dementia.* Nursing and Residential Care, 3 (12): 586-589.

Post, S.G., (1995) The Moral Challenge of Alzheimer Disease. Baltimore, MD: Johns Hopkins University Press.

Rice, T., (2003) *From 'Smart' Homes to 'WISE' Homes.* Journal of Dementia Care, 11 (11) 5.

Roszak, T., (1994) The Cult of Information. Berkeley: University of California Press.

Skolimowski, H., (1983) *The structure of Thinking in Technology.* In Mitcham, C., & Mackey, R., (eds.) Philosophy and Technology: Readings in the philosophical problems of technology. New York: The Free Press.

Staudenmaier, J.W., (1985) *Technology's Storytellers.* Cambridge, MIT Press.

Tunstall Group., (2003) *Project review: Safe at Home Project.* Available from: http://www.tunstall.co.uk (Accessed February 2005).

Winner, L., (2004) *Technologies as Forms of Life.* In Kaplan, D.M. (ed.) Readings in the Philosophy of Technology. Lanham: Rowman and Littlefield Publishers.

Woolham, J., & Frisby, B., (2002) *HowTechnology can help People Feel Safe at Home.* Journal of Dementia Care, 10 (2): 27-29.

7. Assistive technology for people with dementia: legal aspects

Michael Mandelstam

Introduction. Nobody seems to doubt that assistive technology has the potential to be very useful in helping to care for people living with dementia. Nevertheless, it appears that legal concerns sometimes cast into doubt the decision whether to, and when to, use it. Yet law is not the obstacle to creative use of assistive technology that some people suppose. At the same time, the law can – and should - act as a brake on its inappropriate use.

This chapter provides a selective overview of the law underlying the provision of assistive technology for people with dementia. Its purpose is to show how law can be used to underpin good practice.

There is a considerable amount of relevant law. In order to keep the chapter manageable, only a broad summary is given. Examples are used to illustrate some of the practical implications.

The chapter divides the legal framework into the following areas of law:

i. Provision by local social services authorities
ii. Provision by housing authorities: home adaptations
iii. Provision by the NHS
iv. Human rights
v. Disability discrimination
vi. Decision-making capacity and informed consent.
vii. Health and safety at work
viii. Negligence

i. Provision by local social services authorities

i.i. Assessment of need. Local authority social services departments in England and Wales have a specific duty to assess any person aged 18 years or over who appears to be in need of community care services (NHS and Community Care Act 1990, s.47).

In addition, a disabled person has a right to assessment of his or her need for services under the *Chronically Sick and Disabled Persons Act 1970* – if this is requested by the person or his or her informal carer (see s.4 of the *Disabled Persons (Services, Consultation and Representation) Act 1986)*. People with dementia are clearly covered by these duties.

Note. The equivalent to s.47 of the NHS and Community Care Act 1990 in Scotland, is s.12A of the Social Work (Scotland) Act 1968. In Northern Ireland there is no equivalent. In addition, the 1986 Act applies in Scotland, as does the 1970 Act by virtue of the *Chronically Sick and Disabled Persons (Scotland) Act 1972*. The equivalent duties in Northern Ireland come under the *Chronically Sick and Disabled Persons (Northern Ireland) Act 1978* and the *Disabled Persons (Northern Ireland) Act 1989*. The equivalent in Northern Ireland of social services local authorities are health and social services trusts; in Scotland, local authority social work departments are the equivalent of social services departments in England and Wales.

i.ii. Community care services: including assistive technology. Community care services in England and Wales are defined by reference to a number of pieces of legislation additional to the *NHS and Community Care Act 1990*. In other words, the assessment duty is in the 1990 Act, but the actual services lie in other Acts of Parliament.

The service user groups covered in these Acts include those with a mental disorder and therefore people with dementia. The relevant Acts in

England and Wales are Part 3 of the *National Assistance Act 1948, Chronically Sick and Disabled Persons Act 1970 (s.2), Health Services and Public Health Act 1968 (s.45), NHS Act 1977* (schedule 8), and *Mental Health Act 1983* (s.117). Under this legislation, a wide range of services is potentially available, in residential and non-residential settings. Services can include assistive technology. In certain circumstances local authorities might be under a duty to provide assistive technology if this is the only way of meeting an assessed, eligible need.

Example: policy not to provide cheaper items of assistive technology. A local authority has a policy not to provide any items of equipment or assistive technology costing under £50.00. This policy is then applied to a person with dementia, whose assessment by the local authority has revealed an otherwise eligible need for a range of smaller items such as timer-operated medication dispenser, day and night/calendar clocks, smoke detector, heat detector, carbon monoxide detector etc. Each of these costs under £50.00 when taken in isolation and so will not supplied by the local authority.

This policy may be unlawful insofar as it is rigid and represents a `fettering of discretion'; and because it prevents the local authority from meeting the person's assessed, eligible, needs (where the person is in no position to arrange the provision of these items herself).

Example: policy not to spend more than a certain amount on assistive technology. A local authority has a policy that it will spend only up to a total of £1000.00 on assistive technology

for a person with dementia in his or her own home. Such a policy may be unlawful if it is applied rigidly; again because it would fetter the local authority's discretion. It would also prevent it meeting the needs of people for whom placement in a care home would not be a reasonable way of meeting a person's assessed needs.

Note. Apart from the *Chronically Sick and Disabled Persons Act 1970* and its equivalents (see note above) in Scotland and Northern Ireland, the equivalent community care services in those two countries are to be found in s.12 of the *Social Work (Scotland) Act 1968*, s.25 of the *Mental Health (Scotland) Act 1984* (soon to be superseded by the *Mental Health (Care and Treatment) (Scotland) Act 2003*), *Health and Personal Social Services (Northern Ireland) Order 1972*, and a.112 of the *Mental Health (NI) Order 1986*

i.iii. Breadth of social services assessment: determines technology or other solution. Assessment of need should, legally, be wide in scope. This is a key point, *because the types of solution proposed for people with dementia will be determined by the approach taken in assessment.*

For instance, the courts have held that local authorities must take account of a person's psychological needs (*R v Avon CC, ex p M*), culture and language (*R (Khana) v Southwark LBC*), wishes or preferences (*R v North Yorkshire CC, ex p Hargreaves*). In another case, the court stated that the local authority would have to take account of the emotional, psychological and social impact on the person. This would be in terms of wishes, feelings, reluctance, fear, refusal, dignity, integrity and quality of life (*A&B, X&Y v East Sussex County Council*). It should be noted that this duty to assess widely is irrespective of a person's mental capacity; at least two of these cases (*Southwark* and *East Sussex*) involved people potentially lacking the capacity to decide about their care and assistance.

> **Example: assistive technology or personal contact**. A person with dementia lives with her frail husband. He does his best to care for her. She also receives regular visits and assistance from social services staff. Following a review of her needs, the care manager considers whether to install sensors and an alarm and to withdraw some of the visits. The care manager notes that the woman responds very positively to additional human company, and regards this as part of her assessed need. Therefore, in order that the local authority ensures that her assessed needs are met, he decides not to reduce the visits.

i.iv. Social services assessment: risk to independence. 'Fair access to care' guidance issued by central government in England and Wales states that people's needs should be assessed in terms of level of risk to independence (LAC(2002)13; WHC(2002)32). The guidance stresses a wide range of factors that should be considered, going far beyond simple physical risk. Included are matters such as social and family roles and responsibilities, distress, disruption, autonomy and freedom to make choices, daily routines, leisure, hobbies etc.

Assessment of risks to independence is not simply about risk removal or elimination. The provision of services and assistive technology is often about striking a balance between levels of risk and benefits to the service user. For instance, in some circumstances a higher level of risk will be justified if it is balanced by the benefits accruing from that risk.

These same principles apply in relation to people with dementia. Furthermore, it should not be assumed that simply because a person has dementia that they cannot take any decisions and understand certain issues of risk. Decision-making *capacity* may vary from person to person and from issue to issue.

i.v. Social services assessment and joint working with the NHS. Even where 'joint working' takes place between social services and the NHS in England, Wales and Scotland, the duty to carry out a wide-ranging assessment remains. In other words, care must be taken that this social services duty of assessment – whether of a person with dementia or of anybody else - is not diminished in the name of joint working.

Note. In Scotland, joint working provisions come under the *Community Care and Health (Scotland) Act 2002*. In Northern Ireland, there is no equivalent; health and social services already come together in health and social services boards and trusts.

i.vi. Absolute duty to meet assessed, eligible need. Most local authorities apply criteria of eligibility in order to decide whether a person's needs are sufficient to warrant assistance and service provision.

For example, in England and Wales local authorities define people's needs in terms of critical, substantial, moderate and low levels of risk to independence (LAC(2002)13; WHC(2002)32). Each local authority then sets a threshold of eligibility, above which services will be provided and below which they will not. The threshold is set in different places in different authorities. Sometimes the same authority will change the threshold from year to year.

However, once a person has been assessed and found to have an eligible need, the local authority has an absolute duty, irrespective of resources, to meet that need one way or another and without undue delay. Nevertheless if there is more than one option to meet the need, then the local authority may offer that cheaper option but only if it genuinely meets the assessed need (and is consistent with human rights) (e.g. *R v Lancashire CC, ex p RADAR*). The following examples illustrate this point and also that care should be taken to avoid the inappropriate use of assistive technology.

Example: personal assistance or technology? A person living alone with dementia receives support from social services. This includes accompanied walks to local shops to do the food and other shopping. The care plans states that these trips are highly beneficial to him, meeting needs for exercise and social interaction.

In due course a reassessment of the person is completed. The local authority is particularly keen to make use of new technology and one of its local targets is to assist people to use internet shopping. It therefore proposes that he be assisted to do internet shopping from home; this will be quicker and cheaper than accompanying him to the shops.

However, while such a solution would meet the man's need for food, it would not meet his assessed need for social interaction and exercise. Therefore, though cheaper, internet shopping in this case would not alone be capable of lawfully meeting the man's assessed need.

Example: options to meet need: care home, personal assistance, assistive technology? A social services care manager reviews the possible options for a care plan for a man with dementia living at home. The alternatives are two or three visits a day by care staff, seeking admission into residential care, or the use of a passive and active alarm system linked either to a neighbour or to a call centre.

Placing him in a care home is ruled out because it would be likely to distress him greatly. He has indicated very clearly in the past and recently, that he wishes to remain in his own home. Relying on a neighbour to respond to any alarm system is also excluded, since the neighbour, though willing, is frail herself and does not feel able to accept this role. It is finally decided that both an active/passive alarm system linked to a call centre and some visits by care staff represent the best solution. Though more expensive than using technology alone, the visits represent important social contact for this man.

i.vii. Carers. Where informal carers provide care on a regular and substantial basis and request an assessment, local authorities in England and Wales have a duty to assess the ability of such carers to provide care (*Carers (Recognition and Services) Act 1995, Carers and Disabled Children Act 2000, Carers (Equal Opportunities) Act 2004*). Local authorities also have a duty under the 2000 Act to decide whether to provide services for a carer in his or her own right.

Quite clearly, the decision as to whether to provide assistive technology may relate directly to the carer. This might either be a service for the carer, or one for the cared for person that also benefits the carer (as in the following example).

> **Example: carer not sleeping**. A woman has had many interrupted and sleepless nights. Her husband with dementia sleeps in a separate bedroom but is prone to get up during the night. His safety is at risk. She receives a carer's assessment from social services and explains that she cannot go on like this. Social services provide a device that is attached to the husband's bedroom doorwhich, when opened during the night, sets off a quiet alarm by the wife's bedside. This enables her to relax and sleep at night knowing that she will be awakened if he gets up and leaves his bedroom. (From a legal point of view, either he consents to this arrangement or, if he is unable to consent, then it would have to be argued that this arrangement would be in his best interests).

Note. The equivalent carers' provisions elsewhere in the United Kingdom are to be found in the *Social Work (Scotland) Act 1968* (though without provision for carers' services) and in the *Carers and Direct Payments (Northern Ireland) Act 2002*.

i.viii. Community care direct payments. If certain conditions are met, local authorities have a duty to make direct payments for non-residential community care services. A direct payment enables service users, following assessment of eligible need, to purchase their own services - or assistive technology - rather than have them arranged by the local authority.

The conditions for a direct payment are basically as follows.
- The person must (be able to) consent and be able to manage (i.e.

control) the payment with or without assistance.
- The service or equipment in question must meet the assessed need.

Assumptions should not be made about a person's ability to consent and to manage the payment with or without assistance; nor should a local authority apply a blanket policy about what type of service user is eligible for direct payments. To do so would be to put the authority at risk of breaching the direct payments legislation, and of unlawfully 'fettering its discretion' by applying an excessively rigid policy.

If a person with dementia is clearly unable to consent to, or to manage the payment, even with assistance, there is an alternative. This would be for the local authority to make what is variously referred to as a third party or *indirect* payment or a 'user independent trust'. In England or Wales, the courts have identified that such a payment may be made under s.30 of the *National Assistance Act 1948*.

If a person takes a decision to receive direct payments and then loses capacity through dementia, it has been suggested in Department of Health guidance that a person with enduring power of attorney could continue to receive the payments until a reassessment or review is carried out and services changed, at which point the attorney could no longer receive the payments. Thus, initially continuing to receive the direct payments might legitimately be regarded as a financial matter. But once a change in service occurs it would be a welfare matter and beyond the authority of attorney (Department of Health (2003). *Direct payments guidance: community care, services for carers and children's services (direct payments) guidance England 2003).*

The position is different in Scotland where, for people lacking capacity, a welfare attorney or guardian appointed under the *Adults with Incapacity (Scotland) Act 2000*, could take decisions about direct payments: (see s.7 of the *Community Care and Health (Scotland) Act 2002).*

It should be noted that the *Mental Capacity Act 2005* for England and Wales, when in force, will replace enduring power of attorney with lasting power of attorney. The latter would extend not just to business, property and finance but *also* to health and welfare. This would mean a person with a lasting power of attorney would potentially be able to take a decision about direct payments, both initially to receive them and to continue to do so.

Note. Direct payments in England and Wales are covered by the *Health and Social Care Act 2001*. The equivalent legislation in Scotland is to be found in the *Social Work (Scotland) Act 1968*; and in Northern Ireland in the *Carers and Direct Payments (Northern Ireland) Act 2002*.

i.ix. Social services charges for assistive technology. In England and Wales, local authorities generally have a power, although not a duty, to make charges for non-residential services. Any charge must be a reasonable one. If satisfied that it is not reasonably practicable for the person being charged to pay it, the local authority must reduce the charge (*Health and Social Services and Social Adjudications Act 1983).*

In England, however, local authorities are not permitted to charge for any equipment they provide (at whatever cost), or for adaptations costing under £1000.00. This is under the *Community Care (Delayed Discharges) Qualifying Regulations 2003* (SI 2003/1196).

Note. In Scotland, local authorities have a power to charge for non-residential services under s.87 of the *Social Work (Scotland) Act 1968*. The charge must be reasonable and not more than it is reasonably practicable for the person to pay. However, this power does not extend to services that are deemed to amount to personal care under s.1 of the *Community Care and Health (Scotland) Act 2002*. It is notable that that most equipment and adaptations are not classed as coming within personal care.

However, the Scottish legislation expressly includes memory and safety devices as coming within personal care. Guidance refers to such devices which help individuals to manage their own personal care needs – such as personal reminder systems for taking medicine, sound/movement alarms linked to light controls to guide people with dementia to the toilet and to minimise the risks related to wandering at night. Nevertheless, community alarms and other associated devices are not included within free personal care (*Community Care and Health (Scotland) Act 2002*, schedule 1; and see also Circular CCD 4/2002, *Implementation of free personal care and nursing care: guidance*).

Additional Scottish guidance states that frail older people leaving hospital should not be charged for equipment and minor adaptations provided by local authority social work services, if these are supplied and fitted within a four week period following - or immediately prior to, and in preparation for - the hospital discharge (Circular CCD2/2001: *Free home care for older people leaving hospital*).

In Northern Ireland, the power to make an appropriate charge for social services comes under a.15 of the *Health and Personal Social Services (Northern Ireland) Order 1972*.

ii. Provision by housing authorities: home adaptations

Apart from exercising social services functions, local authorities in England, Wales and Scotland also exercise housing functions. In Northern Ireland, housing functions are exercised by the Northern Ireland Housing Executive. Amongst these functions is the provision of home adaptations for disabled people.

Disability as defined for the purpose of home adaptations provided under housing legislation includes mental disorder and therefore includes people with dementia.

In England, Wales and Northern Ireland, housing authorities have a duty to award disabled facilities grants (DFGs) if certain conditions are satisfied. Key conditions include the following.

First, the proposed adaptation must be for a purpose defined in legislation. These purposes relate to the disabled occupant's access to various parts of the dwelling, the use of certain parts of and facilities within the dwelling, and to safety. Second, the housing authority must be satisfied that the adaptation is necessary and appropriate in relation to the person's needs. Third, it must also be satisfied that the adaptation is reasonable and practicable in respect of the age and condition of the dwelling. Even if all these conditions are met and an application for a home adaptation is approved, the housing authority is obliged to apply a means test.

It is beyond the scope of this chapter to set out the home adaptations system in detail. Nevertheless, the safety purpose contained within the DFG legislation may be of particular relevance to people with dementia. Guidance published by central government gives various examples of adaptations relating to safety. Although not specifically concerning people with dementia, the parallel is clear.

Example: home adaptations for safety. Guidance issued on DFGs in England and Wales refers to various types of adaptation for the purpose of safety. These include, for instance, an enhanced alarm system for people with hearing difficulties in connection with cooking, or installation of guards around fires or radiators (DoE 17/96; NAWC 20/02).

Note. In Scotland, housing authorities have a duty to provide home improvement grants under the Housing (Scotland) Act 1987 for certain standard amenities for a disabled person. Otherwise they have a discretion to award such grants for a wide range of purposes – including therefore adaptations for people with dementia. At the time of writing, the Housing (Scotland) Bill 2005 proposes to amend the Scottish system.

iii. Health service provision of assistive technology

Provision of services and equipment by the health service in the United Kingdom is governed by vague legislation. In principle, such provision is governed by duties, but in practice these duties are regarded as so broad and vague that they amount to little more than powers. This means that if the health service fails to provide services for an individual on the grounds that it lacks resources, that provision is not generally legally enforceable by the individual (e.g. *R v Cambridgeshire Health Authority, ex p B*).

Nevertheless, the health service must take serious notice of central government guidance (such as on continuing care: see below) and it should also avoid fettering its discretion – that is applying a blanket policy on assistive technology or indeed anything else.

Such broad duties cut two ways. They appear legally to place few absolute obligations on the health service; but equally their very breadth allows the health service to do a great deal – if it wants to. In other words, were the health service at national or at local level minded to invest heavily in assistive technology for people with dementia, there would be nothing to stop it doing so.

The main relevant legislation comprises the *NHS Act 1977* (ss.1 and 3, England and Wales), *NHS (Scotland) Act 1978* (ss.1,36,37) and the *Health and Personal Social Services (Northern Ireland) Order 1972* (aa.4,5,). Assistive technology must be free of charge if provided through the health service.

In a 2004 investigation in England, the health service ombudsman concluded that a man with Alzheimer's disease living in his own home should have certain elements of his care funded by the NHS (Health Service Ombudsman, Investigation E.22.02-03). It may in some circumstances therefore be arguable that assistive technology required by a person eligible for continuing care should be NHS funded.

iv. Human rights

Since October 2000, the *Human Rights Act 1998* has integrated the *European Convention on Human Rights* into UK law.

The Act and Convention apply *only* to public bodies. For example, if a relative were to care inappropriately for someone with dementia, that relative would not be in breach of this Act.

As far as people with dementia are concerned, several articles of the Convention are particularly relevant. These include articles 2, 3, 5, 8 and 14.

iv.i. Article 2: right to life. Article 2, covering the right to life, has sometimes been argued (hitherto unsuccessfully) in the context of the closure of care homes:

Example: closing a care home. A local authority closes one of its care homes. A number of people with dementia are moved to another home. Several of them die very shortly afterward. If it could be shown on the evidence that assessment and care planning was poor, and that each of the residents had been at serious and significant risk from the move, then article 2 might be engaged.

Nevertheless, hitherto, no home closures have been successfully resisted in the courts on the basis of article 2, although it has been used in argument.

iv.ii. Article 3: inhuman and degrading treatment. When decisions are taken about how and whether to use assistive technology, inhuman and degrading treatment must be avoided. Generally speaking, the courts set a high threshold for article 3. Thus the circumstances required to breach it must be relatively severe.

Example: restraining people with dementia. The Commission for Health Improvement investigated one NHS mental health trust. It revealed that patients with mental health problems were tied to commodes, fed on them, denied food, clothing and blankets, and so were subjected to abuse - owing to a working culture that allowed unprofessional, counter-therapeutic, degrading and even cruel practices. One matter, about which the Commission was unable to reach a conclusion, concerned allegations that a wooden board and harness, and used for restraint on one of the wards, had been made in the occupational therapy department. (CHI 2000. *Investigation into the North Lakeland NHS Trust.*, London: The Stationery Office). Were such treatment to be scrutinised by a law court, article 3 would almost certainly be in issue.

Example: leaving people in humiliating circumstances. A social services occupational therapist identified a need for accommodation and adaptations for a 48-year old disabled woman (who had suffered a stroke) living with her family and six children. Two years later, the woman's needs remained unmet.

As a consequence, she could not reach the lavatory and soiled herself several times a day, had no privacy, could not go out of the house, could not go upstairs, and could not go anywhere without her husband's assistance. She had to share a cramped living room with her husband and two youngest children; the other children had to go through that room in order to go upstairs. Her husband's health was at risk; his back problem deteriorated. She felt frustrated and humiliated because she was unable to do anything for her family and was totally dependent on them.

The judge found a breach of article 8 (see below) and came close to finding a breach of article 3 (*R v Enfield London Borough Council, ex p Bernard*).

iv.iii. Article 5: deprivation of liberty. Article 5 states that people must not be deprived of their liberty unless this is done according to a procedure prescribed by existing domestic law -

and even then only in particular circumstances.

Example: care home with 'baffle' locks. A person with dementia, lacking the capacity to decide where he wants to live, is placed in a care home. The local authority and his family have agreed that this is in his best interests. The exit doors of the home are effectively locked, in that they have 'baffle' locks, although there are no keys. In other words, the doors are difficult to open. The local authority believes that article 5 is not being breached. First it argues that the doors are not 'locked' in the true sense of the word. Second, even if they are regarded as being locked, and the man is being deprived of his liberty, it is in accordance with the law (best interests/necessity) as he is of unsound mind.

Whether or not the local authority's argument is correct may depend partly on how the local authority can justify the use of the baffle locks - in other words, whether the local authority has genuinely explored less restrictive options, which could include looking at the reasons for the 'wandering', and then exploring other ways of managing any associated risks.

The local authority would have to consider this particularly carefully, in the light of a European Court case in 2004: see note immediately below.

Note: deprivation of liberty and assistive technology The judgment in late 2004 of the European Court of Human Rights, in the 'Bournewood' case (*HL v UK*), raised the question of whether article 5 is currently being breached in the case of significant numbers of people. These are people (including those with dementia) who are being informally 'detained' in hospitals or care homes (as opposed to being detained formally under the Mental Health Act 1983) – but who are unable to consent or dissent to their 'detention' – and who might therefore be deprived of their liberty, because of the degree of control exercised over their daily routines. Department of Health guidance warns that both the NHS and local authorities should review such people and consider whether there are less restrictive ways of accommodating them. If there are not, and the degree of control is such that people are being deprived of their liberty, consideration should be given as to whether formal detention under the Mental Health Act 1983 would be appropriate and legally permissible (Department of Health (2004). *Advice on the decision by the European Court of Human of Human Rights in the case of HL v UK (the Bournewood case)*. This issue is likely to be addressed by a combination of the Mental Capacity Act 2005 and draft Mental Health Bill.

Clearly, the use of assistive technology may in some contexts be part of a routine of close control that amounts to deprivation of liberty; in other contexts, it might enable a loosening of that close control.

iv.iv. Article 8: right to respect for private and family life, home and correspondence. Public bodies are allowed to interfere with this right to respect if certain conditions are met. These conditions are as follows:

- Any such interference must be in accordance with domestic law.
- The interference must be necessary in a democratic society.
- It must be for at least one of a number of purposes. These purposes include the protection of health or morals, protection of the rights and freedoms of other people, and the economic well being of the country.

Therefore, in deciding whether or not article 8 is infringed, public bodies and the courts must perform a balancing act.

Example: interference with home, private and family life. The provision in a person's own home of assistive technology such as sensors is clearly relevant to this right to respect for home, family life and privacy. Likewise, closed circuit television trained on the exits of a care home is arguably an interference with privacy. In which case the question in each case is whether the interference can be justified.

Example: in accordance with the law. Where assistive technology is provided by, for example, a local social services authority, the decision to do so would need to be in accordance with the law. This would mean at the very least that the decision should be taken under the relevant community care legislation, consisting of a lawful, adequate assessment and care plan.

If the person lacks capacity to consent to the assistive technology, then the decision would also need to be consistent with the relevant law concerning decision-making capacity. This would, currently, be the common law of necessity and best interests in England, Wales and Northern Ireland, and in Scotland would be the *Adults with Incapacity (Scotland) Act 2000*.

Example: necessary in a democratic society. The interference by a public body with home, private and family life must be proportionate to the circumstances. In other words, interference should be the least restrictive, whilst still being consistent with the person's welfare or best interests; a sledgehammer should not be taken to crack a nut.

For instance, a care home specialising in dementia care places movement sensors in all the rooms of the residents. These sensors allow staff to know in detail what people are doing within their own rooms. However, the placing of the sensors is not dependent on individual risk assessment, and the residents of the home vary greatly in relation to their respective abilities and the risk they are at day to day.

It would therefore be arguable in respect of any one individual resident (e.g. one at relatively less risk) that the interference with his or her privacy could not be shown to be necessary. This would be a) because of the lack of individual risk assessment, and b) where an individual resident's abilities and level of risk did not in fact justify such intrusion.

Example: protection of a person's health. Closed circuit television is used to monitor the exits from the common parts of a local authority care home. The home justifies this interference with privacy as being for the protection of the residents' health. Nevertheless, it would also have to justify this as being in accordance with the law and 'necessary', i.e. the least restrictive intervention consistent with the welfare of residents.

Example: economic well being of the country. A local authority is contemplating increasing its use of assistive technology, in particular a range of sensors, in order to safeguard the welfare of people with dementia living in their own homes. One of the reasons for doing this is to save money since it believes that visits by care staff will be fewer.

For this to be lawful, the local authority would at the very least have to argue in each individual case that the assistive technology genuinely meets the person's assessed, eligible needs. This is because the courts have stated that a local authority can offer the cheaper of two alternatives for meeting need – so long as that cheaper option does indeed meet the assessed need (*R(Rowe) v Walsall Metropolitan Borough Council; R (Khana) v Southwark London Borough Council*).

iv.v. Article 14: discrimination. Article 14 concerns discrimination. The list of grounds contained in the article fails to include explicitly age or disability. However, the grounds are illustrative only; therefore age and disability are implicitly included. To mount an arguable case in relation to people with dementia, two main hurdles would need to be overcome.

First, an appropriate comparison is required. It would need to be shown that, for example, a local authority or the health service was treating less favourably a person with dementia compared to another person without dementia. Alternatively, it might need to be argued that a person with dementia was being treated less favourably on grounds of age. For instance, a ground of discrimination on the basis of age may exist if older people with dementia were to receive a markedly lower standard of service than younger adults with dementia.

Second, article 14 cannot be argued in isolation. It must be argued in tandem with one of the other articles in the Convention.

v. Disability Discrimination Act 1995

It is unlawful under the Disability Discrimination Act 1995 to discriminate against a disabled person by not providing a service that is provided to others, or providing it on worse terms or at a lower standard than it would be provided for others. The Act also makes it unlawful not to make reasonable adjustments to practices, policies, procedures or in relation to the physical environment or to fail to take reasonable steps to provide auxiliary aids or services where these are needed.

Discrimination means less favourable treatment for a reason relating to a person's disability, or a failure to take reasonable steps such that it is impossible or unreasonably difficult for the disabled person to use the service.

However, less favourable treatment can be justified on grounds of
- health and safety,
- the incapacity of the person to enter into a contract,
- the service provider otherwise being unable to provide the service to the public,
- enabling the service provider provide the service to the disabled person or other members of the public.

These are only justified if the service provider believed that one of these defences applied, and that it was reasonable for the provider to believe this.

Example: policy for people with dementia. A local authority imposes a blanket policy that any person with dementia cannot be taken on outings unless accompanied by two staff. This means that many outings do not take place because of the unavailability of staff. The justification given for this policy is health and safety; however, it has been imposed without any risk assessment having been carried out. The imposition of this policy could constitute disability discrimination since a) it has not been imposed in respect of service users with different types of disability, and b) in respect of any one particular person, there would be no evidence (in terms of risk assessment) to support the health and safety ground as justification for the less favourable treatment.

Unlike the *Human Rights Act 1998*, the DDA applies both to public bodies and to the independent and private sector. However, in comparison with the *Human Rights Act*, an arguable case under the DDA has to show that the discrimination in question relates to disability. Other discriminatory factors are irrelevant.

Example: transferring people with dementia. A local authority imposes lower financial ceilings on home care packages (including assistive technology) for people with dementia than for other groups of service users. Apart from breaches of various other law, the local authority might be breaching the DDA.

Example: older and younger adults with dementia. A local authority generally treats younger adults with dementia more favourably than older adults, in terms of how it assesses need and provides service. However, the reason for this apparent discrimination appears to be based primarily on age and not on disability. If so, a case could probably not so easily be brought under the DDA.

vi. Decision-making capacity and informed consent.

The provision of assistive technology for a person with dementia sometimes causes legal anxiety amongst providers - in particular where it invades privacy and the person concerned lacks capacity to decide whether to have the technology.

With the exceptions of compulsory detention under mental health legislation and removal of people from their homes in certain circumstances (s.47 of *the National Assistance Act 1948* (England, Wales, Scotland; a.37 of the *Health and Personal Social Services (Northern Ireland) Order 1972*), health and welfare decision making for adults lacking capacity takes place under the common law of necessity and best interests (England, Wales and Northern Ireland). In Scotland, the *Adults with Incapacity (Scotland) Act 2000* applies.

vi.i. Consent. At present in England, Wales and Northern Ireland, nobody has an automatic legal right to consent, or to withhold consent, to health or welfare interventions on behalf of adults lacking the capacity to take that decision for themselves.

A decision about whether a person lacking capacity should have assistive technology is taken in that person's best interests. This is because a person with an enduring power of attorney can take decisions on behalf of a person lacking capacity – but only in relation to business, property or finance matters (*Enduring Powers of Attorney Act 1985; Enduring Powers of Attorney (Northern Ireland) Order 1987*). So

the decision to install assistive technology in the home of a person with dementia would in principle be beyond the attorney's power. However, paying for the technology would not be. The position is the same for receivers appointed by the Court of Protection in England and Wales (*Mental Health Act 1983*) or controllers appointed by the High Court in Northern Ireland (*Mental Health (Northern Ireland) Order 1986*).

However, the Mental Capacity Act 2005 for England and Wales will (when it is in force) provide for a form of 'consent' (in the form of proxy decision making) to be given or withheld by a person with a lasting power of attorney, or by a deputy appointed by the Court of Protection. Alternatively, under the new Act, and if such formal powers are not required, carers and professionals will also be able to make such decisions in a person's best interests, if they so in good faith.

Note. In Scotland, guardians or welfare attorneys with the appropriate powers are able to give or withhold such consent in relation to health and welfare decisions under the *Adults with Incapacity (Scotland) Act 2000*.

vi.ii. Watershed between capacity and incapacity to decide. Legally, there is a significant watershed between capacity and incapacity to make a decision. In other words, many legal consequences flow depending on the factor of capacity. The question of whether a person has capacity to take a decision is ultimately a legal one; the route to the answer is a medical one.

The courts take the approach that, unless it can be shown otherwise, capacity (rather than incapacity) should be assumed. Furthermore, capacity is not 'all or nothing'; a person may be capable of taking some decisions but not others.

The courts also take a 'functional' approach to capacity. Roughly speaking the approach to be taken is whether a person can take in information, retain it, weigh it up, understand the consequences and reach a decision. The functional approach is in contrast to the 'status' or 'outcome' approach, which would base a decision about a person's capacity on either the person's mental health status ('he has dementia'), or on the consequences of the decision (i.e. an 'irrational' outcome).

Example: choosing to remain at home. A person with dementia has been in hospital with a broken leg. She wishes emphatically to return home. A hospital occupational therapist believes that she will be at significant risk if she does so. She also believes that the woman lacks capacity to decide this a) because of her status (she has dementia) and b) because of the likely risk-laden consequences of her decision.

However, a physiotherapist points out that this is the wrong way to look at capacity; what the professionals should be doing is to consider whether she understands the decision in question and its consequences. The physiotherapist believes that the woman does have this capacity and explores with a social worker how the risk at home could be *managed* through care staff and assistive technology.

vi.iii. Communication. The law emphasises the importance of making all practicable efforts to communicate with a person before concluding that he or she does not have capacity.

Example: hearing impairment. Staff on an NHS hospital ward are talking to a person with dementia about whether she wants to go home and, if so, what arrangements (including assistive technology) might need to be in place. The staff are about to conclude that the person probably lacks capacity because she is not responding, when a physiotherapist reminds them that the woman is extremely hard of hearing.

vi.iv. Best interests or welfare. The common law test of best interests (or, in Scotland, benefit, under the *Adults with Incapacity (Scotland) Act 2000*) involves roughly

- understanding the past and present wishes of someone with dementia and factors they would have considered;
- encouraging the person to participate as fully as possible in decisions;
- the views of other people whom it is appropriate and practical to consult with about best interests; and
- intervening in the least restrictive way.

The Mental Capacity Act 2005 for England and Wales, when it is in force, will apply a similar approach.

Example: past and present wishes, family views. A local authority is consulting with a woman about her husband's best interests. He has dementia and now lacks the capacity to take decisions about everyday activities. However, he clearly loves exercise and getting out of the house and indicates his wish to do this. His wife is loath to `lock' him in; the local authority is also concerned that this could represent an over-restrictive solution. They decide that they will put a sensor on the front door so that both the wife and a neighbour will know when he leaves the house. He is aware of traffic and they also spend a week going out with him on his walks, pointing out particular landmarks to him, so as to reduce the chance of him becoming lost. The wife is happy that this solution is in her husband's overall best interests. The local authority likewise is satisfied, and also believes that it represents a justifiable balancing of risk and benefit.

Example: assistive technology or human contact? A local authority is discussing with a woman with dementia and her family about how to meet her needs in her own home. She lacks the capacity to take the relevant decisions for herself. One of the issues is whether passive alarm sensors should be used in the home, or whether she would benefit from reasonably frequent visits by care staff.

The family points out that she has always been to some extent 'anti-social', enjoying her own company and being averse to invasions of her privacy. This pattern of behaviour is evident even now. The family suggests therefore that perhaps the assistive technology, with fewer visits, would be in her best interests.

vii. Health and safety at work legislation

vii.i. Duties to employees. Under section 2 of the *Health and Safety at Work Act 1974*, an employer has various duties to employees that relate to ensuring safety and welfare, systems of work, instruction, training, information, supervision and so on. The duties are qualified in that they are to be performed as far as is reasonably practicable.

Duties are also owed to employees under the *Management of Health and Safety at Work Regulations 1999*.

Key duties are therefore governed by the term 'reasonable practicability'. Traditionally, the legal test is to weigh up the level of risk to employees in terms of likely *incidence* and *consequence* – against the cost of doing something about the risk. The courts have stated that reasonable practicability does not demand that an employer spend disproportionate resources on dealing with a low risk. However, in respect of public services, the courts have recognised that the utility or benefit to the public (i.e. service users) of a task or activity must also bear on what is reasonably practicable. In other words, there needs to be a balancing of risk and benefit when implementing a system of work designed to deliver public services but at the same time protect employees from unacceptable risk.

Example: balancing risk to staff with welfare of a person with dementia. A woman with dementia lives in her own home in a town centre location. She sometimes leaves the house at an inappropriate time and inappropriately dressed for the weather. In winter, the woman would be at great risk of hypothermia or even death. At other times there is a risk of her being harmed by traffic or other persons.

To help manage these risks the local authority fits a passive infra-red sensor to the front door which alerts the authority's call care centre by means of a care-line telephone. As there are no relatives or neighbours who are able to help, this results in a rapid response by mobile warden services. The location of this person's dwelling and the times at which she leaves the house create a situation in which the warden (an employee of the local authority) herself is placed in a potentially vulnerable situation. The local authority manages this additional risk by offering a panic alarm to the warden, ensuring that, where possible, visits made at certain times are by two people.

The Health and Safety Executive can bring criminal prosecutions under health and safety at work legislation.

vii.ii. Duty to non-employees. In addition to the duty toward employees (which anyway includes consideration of the needs of non-employees), are explicit duties toward non-employees, some of which are likewise governed by the term 'reasonably practicable'.

The first comes under s.3 of the *Health and Safety at Work Act 1974*. It is a duty, so far as reasonably practicable, to ensure that non-employees are not exposed to risks to their health and safety. The second duty relates to risk assessment under r.3 of the *Management of Health and Safety at Work Regulations 1999*. As with the duties to employees, context is important and will involve a weighing up of risk, costs and benefits.

Example: placing cheap contracts with third party call centre. A local authority contracts with an independent call centre to respond to alarms that are set off by sensors provided for people with dementia. When it placed the contract, the local authority allocated relatively very little money to the contract. It failed to check on the background and credentials of the call centre and failed to monitor the performance of the contract. After two serious accidents to service users, attributable to the non-response of the call centre, the Health and Safety Executive decides to investigate whether there has been a breach by both the call centre and the local authority of s.3 of the 1974 Act.

The Health and Safety Executive (HSE) recognises that care packages set up by local authorities may involve 'elective' risk taking. In case of things going wrong, the HSE would not necessarily object to a care package including elements of risk for the service user. Rather it would look to see whether the local authority's risk assessment and care plan were adequate and had sufficiently balanced the benefits and wishes of the service on the one hand, with the risks on the other (HSE SIM 7/2000/08. *Social services social inclusion and elective risk*).

viii. Negligence

The common law of negligence applies a basic test of

- whether harm has been caused to a person,
- how it was caused,
- whether it was caused by carelessness (i.e. a failure to take *reasonable* care), and
- whether the careless person or organisation owed a duty of care in the particular context.

The test of 'reasonableness' is similar to that for 'reasonable practicability' under health and safety work legislation. It, too, involves weighing up risk against the cost of doing something about it. In the case of public bodies such as local authorities, it will also include consideration of benefits to service users.

In addition to the relevance of the law of negligence to product use and safety, is the *Consumer Protection Act 1987*. Part 1 of this Act places what is in principle strict civil liability on manufacturers whose products are defective and cause harm. There are some defences available to the manufacturer, including one relating to whether the manufacturer could have been expected to discover the defect at the time of manufacture.

Example: purchase of sensors. A local authority purchases and provides a range of sensors for people with dementia. However, rather than purchase on the basis of genuine 'best value' or cost effectiveness, it has simply purchased the cheapest. They are of doubtful quality, contain poor instructions, and have failed on a number of occasions. Nevertheless, the local authority persists in using them. There are several incidents of concern. There is then a fatality arguably attributable to the failure of one of the sensors. The dead person's family considers whether to sue both the manufacturer under the *Consumer Protection Act 1987* and also the local authority in negligence.

Example: using assistive technology for an alternative purpose? A local authority wonders whether to use burglar alarms that work on the sensor principle to assist with the care of people dementia. It is concerned

that it is using equipment for an ultimate purpose not originally intended by the manufacturer. However, the equipment would perform the same function intended by the manufacturer, namely detection of movement. It is just the context and response that would differ. *Therefore, so long as the local authority had satisfied itself that the alarms were fit for the purpose it intended (detecting movement with sufficient reliability in the context of potentially life threatening situations))*, it is unlikely that there would be any particular legal problems (all other things being equal).

Example: using assistive technology in a different way. In contrast to the example immediately above, assistive technology might be used not just in a different context, but in a completely different way. There is no law against doing this, but clearly the risks may become greater and will require careful assessment. An example of what can go wrong occurred when tongue depressors were used as limb splints in a neonatal intensive care unit. Fungal infection caused by the depressors resulted in two deaths and one amputation (referred to in: MDA/2004/006: *medical devices in general and non-medical products*).

Example: installation of equipment. A local authority and the NHS jointly fund a range of sensors in the homes of a number of people with dementia. They have a contract with an independent company to install them. The sensors fail in several cases, causing harm to the service users concerned. On investigation it appears that the sensors were of good quality and were supplied with clear instructions. However, the installation process had been carelessly undertaken. A negligence case might lie against the installer, and also against the local authority and NHS if it could be shown that they had not paid due care to the setting up and monitoring of the contract.

ix. Conclusion.

This chapter has set out a number of different areas of law. Overall, it has outlined the following.

First, statutory services, particularly local authorities, have potentially strong obligations to meet the needs of people with dementia by means of assistive technology. However, this must involve using assistive technology genuinely to meet assessed need rather than simply as a cheaper alternative to care that does not properly meet an assessed need.

Second, use of assistive technology is not inconsistent with human rights, but the Human Rights Act 1998 offers important safeguards against the misuse of such technology.

Third, health and safety at work legislation and the law of negligence emphasise the principles of 'reasonable practicability' and 'reasonableness'. These principles are not inimical to the use of assistive technology for people with dementia or, indeed, with the taking of risks. They *do* require that due care be taken and, where risks are in issue, that an adequate balancing of risk and benefit (to the service user) has taken place.

In conclusion, the law does not support the use of assistive technology for people with dementia where it does not genuinely meet assessed needs or places people at undue risk. Nor does it demand the type of defensive and anxious decision-making which would hinder the positive use of such technology. Instead the law arguably demands a balanced approach, which in turn is most likely to support good practice.

8. 'Working in the Zone' - A Social -Ecological framework for dementia rehabilitation

Stephen Wey

As a practitioner my interest in assistive technology has always been to see it as an aspect of a rehabilitative and enabling approach. I have a real concern at the moment that as interest in assistive technology takes off (and it seems to me that it is taking off now, and some powerful drivers have become interested in its potential) the human element in the provision of such technology could get increasingly left out. Here is an example. A few years ago I was asked to assess a gentleman on a medical ward who was falling a lot. He had experienced something like 17 falls in one week. As a result of my assessment one of the recommendations I made was the use of a sensor mat placed on his chair to inform nursing staff of when this gentleman got up. At that time, such technology was fairly new. However I also made clear as part of my recommendations that the use of this sensor mat must be married to a care plan that would ensure that when a nurse responded to the sensor mat going off, this gentleman would not be simply told to sit down again but would be asked what he wanted. Did he want the toilet? To go for a walk? To stretch his legs? The human element. Simple good practice, but without this such technology would become disabling, not enabling. So, for me, provision of assistive technology for a person with dementia must be considered within the context of a person-centred, social model of rehabilitation and disability. Without such a model, there is a real danger that technology could be used as a 'quick fix' rather than as a means of improving social inclusion and empowering individuals with dementia. This sort of thinking was briefly explored in an earlier paper (Wey 2004) where such a model was implicit in the decision making process used in selecting person-centred interventions using assistive technology based solutions for people with dementia living in the community. In this paper I compared several "high" and "low" tech interventions used to "manage" the same risk – that of leaving a cooker on unattended. Even though the same risk was present in each of these situations it was possible to demonstrate that the same intervention would not be appropriate in each case – one size did not fit all. A detailed individual assessment had to be made; not just of the presenting risk but also of the person's capabilities, priorities and wishes, to ensure the intervention chosen was appropriate in helping them maintain their autonomy and well being and not just managing the risk.

While this paper is not specifically about assistive technology it aims to develop these themes further describing a theoretical framework for dementia rehabilitation within which assistive technologies and environmental adaptations are but one component. It's largely based on a process of theoretically informed reflection on practice based experiences while working as an occupational therapist as part of an Intensive Home Treatment Team for people with dementia in the community (Wey 2002). The remit of this team was to provide rapid and intensive assessment and treatment - which included both psycho-social interventions and rehabilitation - in order to prevent inappropriate hospital admissions and facilitate earlier and more sustainable discharges (both from mental health and medical wards) for individuals experiencing dementia.

My aim as an occupational therapist has mainly been to find ways to help bring the world back as much as possible within the person's grasp practically, conceptually and meaningfully. This means considering the 'fit' between the person and their environment. For all of us, as we grow as people, we develop a variety of strategies for coping with the various challenges the world places before us and achieving the goals we set ourselves along the way. We do this through a process of adaptation - both adapting ourselves to the environments we live in, for example by developing skills and knowledge, and adapting our environments to better meet our needs, for example by modifying the environment to make it more accessible or by employing technologies that make life simpler. We strive for a 'fit' between the demands of that environment (social and physical) and our own skills and capabilities, so as to be enabled to make the best use of the resources we have available to us (both internal and external). This concept is referred to as 'person-environment fit' (Lawton & Nahemow 1974), and it has important implications for the provision of any sort of adaptations - including assistive technology and telecare as we need to think about whether the changes we propose to carry out are more likely to increase the fit between person and environment (and therefore decrease disability) or increase it, and push the world further away (and therefore increase disability).

I would describe this sort of approach to dementia rehabilitation as *social* and *ecological*. It is *social,* because we are making use of a positive and therapeutic social psychology, particularly the way that the social environment can be structured to support people in maintaining not just their cognitive and functional skills, but their personhood and well-being. There is a particular emphasis on the *situated* and *distributed* nature of human action. People exist within a social, cultural and historical context; their memories, skills and very personhood do not exist in themselves, but in their relationship with this lived context. It is e*cological,* because it is based in a naturalistic and contextualised process of assessment and enablement. We need to observe people as they function in their own settings, what they do with their living space and their time, how they approach activities and what is meaningful and habitual to them. We should seek to introduce enhancements that work within this context and with the person, primarily with the aim of maintaining personhood, meaningfulness and agency rather than skills *per se*, helping them to make best use of their inner resources and those available to them in the social/physical environment.

One of the big advances proposed by Tom Kitwood and developers of the person-centred approach is that we should understand dementia as a disability; that is within its social, cultural and historical context, and not as reducible to a set of impairments caused by a disease process. If we view dementia from the perspective of a social model of disability, then it falls upon us not just to counter the prevalent 'malignant' social psychology that invalidates and disables people with dementia, but to understand how a positive social psychology can be enabling and empowering. In other words we need a *social model of ability* too. To me that is the essence of a therapeutic and rehabilitative approach to dementia. Kitwood argued that part of the experience of ill-being in dementia may be that:

'everything is falling apart, nothing gets completed, nothing makes sense'

Kitwood, (1990: p. 40-56).

In my view this statement serves as a starting point for a positive approach to rehabilitative and therapeutic practice in dementia care. How can we enable the person to feel supported and validated and to be able to be "held" even through the experience that the world, indeed one's very self, is falling apart, to be enabled to meaningfully complete tasks and activities and continue experience the world as an agent - to be able to say 'I can' and to feel in control over one's life; and to be enabled to make sense of the world and to continue to experience one's own life and being as a person as meaningful and as really counting for something? Influenced in part by the work of the paediatrician DW Winnicott, Kitwood argued that we needed to understand the sort of processes that facilitate the development of the self in childhood if we are to develop a truly therapeutic approach for people at risk of or in the process of losing their own self-hood.

'I think we can summarise Winnicott's position by suggesting that two conditions are absolutely necessary for a young child to acquire a robust and healthy sense of self. The first is an environment of acceptance, love and care, one which is safe enough for the child to experience and work through a whole range of emotions... The infant must somehow come to know that these are part of the

human condition; that experiencing them does not mean that the world is going to collapse; and that love is stronger and more enduring than them all. The second condition is that the young child should develop a sense of agency, of inner vitality, of having the ability to make a mark on others and the world'.

Kitwood, (1993: p.51-67)

Translating this into the context of therapeutic practice for people with dementia I would argue that we need:

i. to provide a holding and validating approach; a 'container' to people who need this when 'everything is falling apart', and
ii. to ensure as much as possible that things to continue to 'make sense' and that the person is enabled to maintain a sense of their own agency and control over their world.

However, where Kitwood drew largely upon Winnicott and attachment theory in outlining a "holding" approach, I found that while offering valuable insights into some of the early attachment processes that form the foundations of the self, Winnicott's theories are perhaps less useful in elucidating the sorts of processes that enable the development of the sense of agency and mastery described under the second condition. In my view a body of theory much closer to forming a "social model" of the development of the self and of agency and mastery in particular was that developed by the Russian psychologist Lev Vygotsky and the later psychologists influenced by his ideas. This is the 'school' of thought sometimes described as 'Social Constructivism' or 'Socially Mediated Activity Theory' (Wertsch 1998).

In order to explore these theories and how they can be applied in practice I would like to try and bring them to life by discussing them in the context of a case study of one person's journey back home from hospital. In this way we will hopefully be able to reflect on some of the process and methods that can facilitate people with dementia in making this transition from hospital care to living their own lives again. So this is Clara's story.

Clara's story

Clara was in hospital for several weeks before our team got involved. She had been admitted following a fall and had recovered fully from a broken hip. At the time the staff on the ward were exploring the option of 24 hour care for Clara as their assessment was that she would be unsafe to return home, even with a package of care. The reasons for this were that on the ward Clara was:

- "Wandersome" - getting lost on the ward and leaving the ward.
- Not responsive to rehabilitation, unable to adapt to using walking aids (a stick) which she needed constant prompting to remember to use,
- therefore she was at risk of falls.
- Unsafe using stairs - Clara lived in a second floor flat and could only get to the door by descending a flight of stairs - although she had been provided with an electronic intercom system she hadn't been able to use it appropriately and the family were concerned she was going to either not let anyone in, or let people in indiscriminately. They also felt she was likely to forget she was at risk of falls and attempt to negotiate the stairs unsafely - she had been unable to retain

attempts to teach her a safer technique on the stairs in hospital.
- Not oriented to day/ time/ place/ person.
- Not always recognising her own family.
- Experiencing a decline in her skills. She'd had a kitchen assessment and had left the cooker on and been unable to cook independently.

At the time, Clara scored 16/30 on a MMSE scale.

Clara was not at all interested in 24 hour care and was anxious to return home as soon as possible. She was becoming low in mood as she felt this would be impossible: she was losing hope day by day. It was painful to watch hope slipping away from her as we felt that given the right conditions and level of support at home Clara would flourish. Her family were supportive of her returning home in principle but were understandably concerned about the risks.

To help provide a "safety net" on Clara's return home and at the same time enable her to allow visitors such as carers and friends access without having to negotiate the stairs she was provided with a monitored intercom system. Access to the front door was controlled by an electronic lock mechanism managed by a 24-hour call centre that could screen visitors based on a list of welcome callers. The centre could also talk to Clara directly to ask if she knew the person at the door. This was important to enable her to retain a 'say so' over access. The system also included an alarm in case she fell or had an emergency, and Clara was able to talk to people at the call centre if she needed help or even someone to talk to.

Clara returned home initially with 3 visits a day from our team, these were reduced to two over the next 2 weeks, then we continued to assess her for another 6 weeks while homecare was gradually introduced. Homecare services were not involved initially as we needed to work with Clara ourselves to determine her range of capabilities, needs and wishes. Ironically, the actions that on the ward had been seen as a problem, we saw as an indication of Clara's potential to adapt. What was construed as being 'wandersome' was an indication she had not become apathetic and withdrawn and was actively trying to make sense of what was happening to her and where she was, as well as seeking out opportunities for occupation and social contact. It is often important to recognise that many such 'behaviours' interpreted as challenging have an adaptive element and flow from the person's need to make sense of things and to communicate their own needs and wishes. Reframing 'challenging behaviour' in this way is not in any sense a question of semantics. It can provide a real handle on opportunities to make therapeutic contact with the person and to start to understand what may be relevant to enabling that individual to maximise their well being. The fact that someone is seeking contact and occupation means that person will probably be motivated to respond to an approach that provides more meaningful occupation and social contact. Making therapeutic contact with the person in this way is the starting point of any meaningful process of assessment and treatment. So what we saw when Clara returned home was a that while she was able to orientate herself once back at home and no longer demonstrated any signs of "wandering," two of the keys to her continued well-being would be social contact and meaningful, manageable occupation.

Clara's pathways - situated cognition and situated personhood.

Many of the things Clara had been unable to do on the ward became understandable when we started to get to know her in her home environment. One of the advantages of working in an intensive home treatment team is that whereas on a hospital home assessment one is limited by pressure to accomplish certain objectives within a very limited space of time, on multiple visits carried out over a few days it becomes possible for assessment processes to be more relaxed and naturalistic. Observations are made within the context of a social visit, or around a shared activity such as making a meal together or walking together, more in the manner of what anthropologists refer to as "participant observation". Every attempt is made to blend in, to use language that is contextual and natural, to be sensitive to the person's culture and biography, and to use approaches such as validation/resolution to build trust and empathy. Therefore it becomes possible to observe in detail how a person functions in their natural setting (which is one of the reasons I refer to this as an "ecological" assessment process) and how that person's functioning is supported or not supported by that setting. Essentially we are trying to understand how the person and their life-world intermesh, how this enables them to maintain their personhood and where it may need to be further augmented, at least for a while, to continue to support that person's well-being. For example, many of the things Clara struggled with while in hospital - remembering to use her stick, recalling family members, knowing the time - took on a new meaning within her home environment. We observed that Clara tended to leave her stick in particular places at home, something she couldn't do in hospital as no place there held the same associations and meanings for her. Memory is like that: it isn't some inert 'recording' - it is lived, sensuous, contextual. A favourite chair may not be just a chair; it may carry memories and associations based on one's life history (which in turn is something that occurs within the context of that person's culture and social history). These rich elements of a person's life-world are not often present in hospital. Furthermore, Clara had "pathways" she generally tended to follow around her flat based on habit patterns, possibly evolved over many years, and she made use of those pathways as a mnemonic aid in the same way I might follow a routine in the mornings to ensure I don't forget to turn off the lights or lock up. So, if she came into the kitchen the radiator was always on her right (she was right handed) and she always hung her stick on the radiator, which meant it was in front of her when she came out again. The second day we visited we became concerned because her medication box had gone missing from where we had left it (in a kitchen cupboard). Clara showed us she had decided to put it under the TV on top of the TV Times. Why, we asked? Because, she said, when she is watching TV she knows what time it is, she used the TV and her TV planner to help her mark time and this also helped her to anticipate when we would visit next. She was an avid "soap" watcher and that really helped her mark time meaningfully. After we'd assessed this for a while it became clear she was able to use this system to self medicate successfully, with an occasional extra prompt only when needed. She also used our visits as a mnemonic, to structure her days,

and she started to write in a notebook she kept next to her, when people were coming, who had visited and sometimes what we did together. Other patterns, such as when the milkman came, family visits etc added to this pattern of life that contained cues for maintaining her memory and skills.

This contextual understanding of thinking and memory is referred to as **'situated cognition'** (Wertsch 1998 & Seely Brown et. al 1989). We all structure our lives and environments in ways (often pre-consciously) that facilitate us in functioning at an optimal level. This is where it's important to consider the degree of "fit" between person and their environment I described above; people adapt themselves to their world and adapt their world to themselves over their whole lifespan. This includes habit patterns and routines, the structure of a room and the objects in it (including significant memories and meanings attached to those objects that help us recall events and feelings), and patterns of activities such as leisure time, personal care time, work time, social contacts. At home Clara's competencies were calibrated to her environment through habitual routines and years of experience. Her level of person-environment fit was much closer to an optimal level for her abilities compared to when she was on the ward.

One could argue that person-hood is itself a situated phenomenon. In many respects it is being *removed* from this structure of socially contextualised activities and routines that deskills people with dementia when they are admitted to hospital. Hospitalisation takes away the meanings and memories that enable such skills and activities to make sense in a practical, applied way (which offers some clues about how ward environments can be made into more therapeutic environments). Clara's memory for people also improved once visits were placed back in a meaningful context. At home visits from family and friends were made within the context of everyday, normalised social life (not hospital visits). In fact we advised the family to notify her when someone was coming and attach visits to a purpose in order to create a familiar structure and routine, whereas in hospital visits were within the context of "hospital time" (not owned by Clara) and within a context that was alien and unfamiliar. I can think of situations myself when I have failed to recognise someone I should have (even people fairly close) due to encountering them in an unfamiliar or unexpected context, (you have to do a "double take" to work out what's amiss, something that requires quite a lot of cognitive capacity and flexibility). Most importantly for Clara, her time was her own. In hospital there were frequent, unscheduled interruptions that made it hard for anyone to establish any meaningful routine. At home she could set her own pace and not be out-paced by her environment and the people in it - ownership of time is an essential feature of well-being and situated personhood.

Distributed cognition and working in "The Zone"

Two areas of rehab with which Clara had particular difficulty when assessed in hospital were in relation to cooking meals for herself and using the stairs safely. In both activities she was felt to be unsafe left to her own devices. However once back at home it soon became clear that both these activities held significant meaning for Clara, that she needed to feel a measure of

independence in at least being able to cook snacks for herself. Although she didn't need to go up and down the stairs as much due to the intercom system, she still wanted to be able to go out when she wanted to and more importantly, wanted to regain her confidence and to feel more in control of her own life: she saw not being able to negotiate the stairs as a symbolic as well as practical barrier. The issue was one of quality of life and autonomy, not just risk or skills.

The approach used to enable Clara to maintain the autonomy she desired was to work collaboratively and interactively with her to help her identify her own goals and range of capability in order to determine how to best support her in living her life as she wished. Given that the ward's assessment had identified certain difficulties in carrying out activities like cooking and mobilising it was important that she was given the right amount of support so as to experience these activities being successfully and safely completed. But how do we determine *the right amount* of support? It was possible that if she were just left to fend for herself, not only would she have been at risk but her confidence, already fragile, would have been further undermined by experiencing failure in carrying out tasks she would have known she could at one time have managed. In fact there were clear signs this had been starting to happen before she went into hospital. This may have been one of the reasons she was so scared about not returning home and why it was affecting her mood and self-esteem. So the aim was to enable the tasks such as cooking snacks, some housework, practice on the stairs etc, to be completed in as 'failure free' and non-threatening a fashion as possible. However, it was also important to be able to identify what she brought to the activity herself. This required an understanding of her range of capabilities, her problem solving process, how she approached each task, what she responded best to and what got in the way, in order to ensure that the amount of support provided was pitched at the right level. Too much support would also undermine her confidence and contribute to a sense that she was not in control of the activity. How do we go about getting the right balance?

When people collaborate in a shared activity, there is a process of socially shared or *'distributed cognition'* (Saloman 1993). Each person contributes something to the overall activity, and if one person has a greater level of capability in one area then they may help support the other in that particular area and visa versa. For example if I am baking a cake with my daughter there is a field of interaction within which one can delineate 3 areas or zones marking our respective contributions. Firstly there will be some things I know she is fully capable of and can take the lead in. This would consist of skills and capabilities she has fully mastered. At the same time there would be some things I know she needs me to manage completely at this stage, particularly when it comes to ensuring the activity is safe for her. Between these two poles there is a zone where we need to work closely together, where skills she has partially mastered but still needs a bit of help with are further honed, or where I can see ways to grade aspects of the task to help her to master it better in future. There are elements where we need to have a dialogue or process of negotiation about how to proceed. This is a dynamic zone where the aim is to provide *just enough but not too much* support in a graded way that can be pulled back as her mastery increases.

This dynamically changing zone was named the *'zone of proximal development'* (or ZPD) by the psychologist Lev Vygotsky. (1978) He argued that understanding how to work with people in this zone was the key to bringing to the surface developing, potential or latent skills and capabilities. We didn't need to just assess what people could (or could not) do independently. We also needed to understand what they were most ready to do, their range of potential and *the circumstances under which that potential could be actualised.* So the zone of proximal development is:

'The distance between the actual developmental level as determined by independent problem solving and the level of potential development as determined through problem solving under adult guidance or in collaboration with more capable peers'

Vygotsky, (1978: p. 78)

Vygotsky's contribution here is his view that the development of the self and of capability is a social and cultural phenomenon, not an individual process of working through a series of intrinsic stages but one where the child is actively supported and encouraged through a process of inclusion in socially shared and mediated activities.

'From the moment of birth, children are in constant interaction with adults who actively seek to incorporate them into their culture and its historically accumulated store of meanings and ways of doing things. In the beginning, children's responses to the world are dominated by natural processes, namely those provided by their biological heritage. But through the constant intercession of

adults, more complex, instrumental psychological processes begin to take shape. At first, these processes can operate only in the course of the children's interaction with adults. As Vygotsky phrased it, the processes are interpsychic; that is, they are shared between people. Adults at this stage are external agents mediating the children's contact with the world. But as children grow older, the processes that were initially shared with adults come to be performed within the children themselves. That is, the mediated responding to the world becomes an intrapsychic process. It is through this interiorisation of historically determined and culturally organised ways of operating on information that the social nature of people comes to be their psychological nature as well.'

Luria, (1979: p. 44)

Furthermore Vygotsky argued that whereas assessment of the child's independent functioning could help reveal their current level of development, it was only in situations where they were enabled to participate in such shared activities that their potential areas of development would emerge. In other words:

'What a child can do with assistance today, she will be able to do by herself tomorrow.'

Vygotsky, (1978: p. 87)

Although he worked largely with children and adults with learning disabilities Vygotsky's model can be applied to explain how the structure of shared activities and social learning environments occurs and develops throughout the human lifespan. For example, Cole writes:

'I would like to treat the idea of a Zone of Proximal Development in terms of its general conception as the structure of joint activity in any context where there are participants who exercise differential responsibility by virtue of differential expertise'.

Cole (1985)

In the context of dementia rehabilitation we also want to help individuals adapt to a changing world. Traditionally, there has been an argument that people with dementia are not suitable for rehabilitation - usually, as the formula goes, because they cannot learn 'new skills'. In fact the whole process of dementia is one of having to adapt, whether one wants to or not, to an often dramatically changing inner and outer world. The question we must ask ourselves is should people have to make those adaptations in an unsupported way? The answer is that we should try to provide a process that facilitates adaptation in a manner that is validating and enabling, and one which seeks to help preserve as much as possible of the meaningfulness of the world for the person with dementia - in particular the sense of being in control and of being an 'agent'. I would also argue that even if we were to leave aside the question of "new" skills (and would question what that term really means as well) we are certainly aiming to help provide the best conditions for bringing out the person's potential, especially skills and capabilities that are becoming less used or latent, or that are no longer fully integrated into the person's repertoire or meaningful social roles.

How we provide a suitably *enabling and facilitatory environment,* where the person is given just the critical amount of support to enable them to complete a task, but not too much, is the key to ensuring the integrity and meaningfulness of such activities. This process is referred to by educational psychologists influenced by Vygotsky (such as Jerome Bruner) as *'scaffolding'*.

Scaffolding may be broadly described (to paraphrase Cole's quote above) as the way a joint activity is structured interactively and dynamically *in any context where there are participants who exercise differential responsibility by virtue of differential expertise* so as to enable the participant who is less able to function at a higher level than they would if they were on their own. Such *"structuring"* may involve simplifying an aspect or aspects of the activity to enable it to be more within the person's grasp (practically or conceptually), it may involve *grading* the level of the task in some way or *pacing* the activity to ensure it is not progressing too fast for it to be manageable. Greenberg-Lyons, a Paediatric occupational therapist describes a number of methods she uses to Scaffold children through an activity.

> *'The process of defining the child's zone of proximal development involves the therapist working on a problem with the child and discovering what support facilitates the child's ability to exhibit emerging cognitive capacities such as attention, perception or problem solving'*

Greenberg Lyons, (1984: p. 446-451).

She describes using the following interventions amongst others:

- Touching stimuli to focus attention
- Altering the size, arrangement and complexity of task components
- Modifying language to make it less abstract (embedded or contextualised)
- Using concrete cues and gestural prompts
- Using motivational techniques (e.g. playfulness, clown's face)
- Co-active physical assistance /prompting

An often cited example would be working with a child on a jigsaw puzzle where the parent (or teacher or more skilled peer) initially completes the edges and the child fills in the middle. Then gradually as and when the child's skill develops the degree of assistance provided and approach is reduced or adapted to their developing needs. However it is important to note that scaffolding is not reducible to any one process or technique: it serves as a model for facilitatory relationships rather than a prescription for one particular method of facilitation. The approach used depends on the individual, the level they are operating at, the overall goal and the context:

> *'Independent problem-solving indicates what cognitive functioning the child has already mastered; problems which the child can only solve with assistance suggest what functions are still immature but are in the process of becoming ready for independent use. There is little point in offering scaffolding below the bottom of the ZPD, because the child can already function here without it, or above the top of the ZPD, because the difference from the child's present functioning may be too great. Within the ZPD, adult-child interaction is likely to facilitate development, though it may do so in a sequence of different*

ways. During the earliest periods of learning in the ZPD, a child may have a very limited understanding of what the task involves; the teacher offers a model or successive precise and simple directions, and the child merely observes or imitates. Gradually, as the child is able to cope with more components of an activity, and has greater understanding of how they fit together - an understanding that includes more appreciation of what the goal is and how best to reach it - the adult reduces the assistance given and changes from very directive help to suggestion and encouragement. The adult needs to take less and less responsibility for the successful performance of the activity as the increasingly competent learner takes it on'.

Meadows, (1996: p. 32).

The focus of Scaffolding is on the structure of the relationship and how it mediates successful performance of the activity. This focus provides the best conditions for helping the person acquire and to maintain a sense of agency in a way that helps preserve the integrity of the activity as a meaningful process: that is to say, skills and competencies are not passed on as abstract entities but within the context of a socially and culturally meaningful activity. The emphasis is not on developing skill *per se*, but on developing and facilitating the person's sense of mastery and agency under conditions where there is support available if things don't work out and a guiding hand to adapt the structuring process dynamically to the individual's needs. Kitwood was aware I think of this sort of process, in its most basic form, when he described the following interaction between parent and child:

'The infant makes a gesture. It may be an incompletely co-ordinated body movement, a cry, a gasp, or the beginning of a little game. The sensitive caregiver sees the gesture and responds to it, destroying nothing of its originality and direction, but helping to fill it out with meaning and make it into an action.

A central hypothesis is that such joint ventures, successfully completed, convey to the infant that he or she is an agent; one whose movements, coming increasingly within conscious control, have meaning, and one whose intentions count for something in the world'.

Kitwood, (1990: p. 40-56).

He also saw such joint ventures as a model for facilitatory practice where the aim is of building agency and maintaining meaningfulness. I see this as an extension of what he described as *holding*, but into the realm of socially mediated action; actions which become a shared process of validation and social inclusion.

'Adults 'scaffold' the child through the task to be carried out, doing the parts the child cannot do and arranging the situation so that the child can take his or her part. They direct attention to currently relevant features of the task; they suggest what might be considered, remembered or done; they model appropriate actions and strategies; they supervise and provide feedback on the child's actions. Adult and child take turns to carry out the steps of the task, with responsibility for its execution gradually shifting from adult to child; the strategies needed for the task are modelled, overtly, again and again, and the

child practices them again and again; the adult gives the child a little more independence after a successful action, and a little more support if there has been a failure or difficulty. The child is helped to progress through the 'zone of proximal development'.

Meadows, (1993: p. 338).

Working with Clara preparing meals or practicing a new technique on the stairs followed an approach influenced by these concepts. The aim was to create an interactive dialogue based around the activity that would create the best conditions for Clara to master the skills required while making the best use of those she already had and maintaining the integrity and overall meaningfulness of the activity.

For example, one goal was to help Clara internalise a safer method of descending the stairs. Realistically we knew that she would continue to try and do this, unless her access to the stairs was blocked off completely - something that would have really impacted on her well-being and autonomy. We had to find a way to help her do this as safely as possible. A minor environmental modification, fitting an additional banister, helped her to balance better, but the key was that she needed to use a technique of descending the stairs one step at a time, leading with her strongest leg, and briefly pause to ensure she was fully balanced before taking the next step. Initially the technique was demonstrated to her rehearsed together with the accompanying verbal cues ("one step, stop") before actually starting down the stairs. At first these were repeated jointly as she began her descent, then after a few steps Clara was allowed to carry on by herself. If it looked like she was starting to lose the thread she would be provided with a shared verbal cue again for a few more steps and then again this would be pulled back. The aim was to help her establish a process of self talk, one that was initially externalised and shared but that through repetition in practice could become internalised. This process of rehearsal and repetition followed a graduated pattern; so as Clara's competence increased the space between verbal cues was lengthened to allow her time to repeat back the commands to herself internally. Combined with Clara's own motivation and the fact that she was back at home (so the activity was more meaningful for her), she was eventually able to assimilate these techniques fully, reaching a point where she no longer needed to repeat the cues out loud to herself.

When Clara's cooking skills were reassessed in her own home it was important to identify Clara's own problem solving process and the way she approached tasks and made use of the cues inherent within the activity and the social and physical environment. Clara often proved to be able to come up with creative solutions when presented with problems (for example, her technique of remembering where to place her pills cited earlier). She was also able to sequence tasks like cooking a simple meal such as bacon and eggs from beginning to end, including locating the materials she needed and was also able to carry out several sub-tasks simultaneously (such as maintaining an eye on a saucepan and a frying pan). One thing that became apparent when working with her was due to having some moderate visual and auditory deficits she had to put more into concentrating on the task in hand and at times this led to her not taking on board feedback from what she was doing, not noticing when something wasn't fully turned off at the end of the activity for example. This wasn't helped by the fact that the cooker was old and the markings on the dials were indistinct. Once we had provided her with some stickers on the cooker clearly marking the on/off positions and provided her with a few clear written cues to ensure everything was off in strategic places she was able to cook light snacks (one pan dishes, toast, porridge) for herself safely.

At this point I feel it would be useful to briefly reflect again on the three case studies (of which Clara was one) presented in "One Size does not fit all" (Wey, 2004). Each person presented in these studies was identified as having the same problem - leaving the cooker on unattended. And yet for each person when looked at in more detail the reasons for them doing this and the solutions chosen were very different. For Mary, a lady for whom a daily routine of shopping and cooking played a central role in maintaining both her personhood and her functional and cognitive abilities, it was clear that the priority was to help her to carry on cooking as long as possible, but to provide a safety net when needed. So she was supplied with a gas sensor that gave out an alarm call if she left the gas on and if it built up to a dangerous level automatically shut off the supply (temporarily). Now one thing that made it possible for such an intervention to work in Mary's case was the frequency of her lapses in skill (which may have been due to a combination of repeated acute infections and possible TIAs or "stepwise" changes). If she had been leaving the gas on everyday for example, or almost every time she attempted to cook, then the disruption in her life caused by having the gas alarm go off and the supply shut off so

frequently could well have negated any benefit derived from enabling her to continue cooking. As it was, Mary's 'lapses' were generally interspaced by several weeks of relative independence and therefore, within a rehabilitative context, such an intervention was well justified as it not only enabled her to maintain those skills, it allowed time for her to accumulate and assimilate any benefits in terms of maintained attention span, stimulation of memory and problem solving skills she would have been deriving from this activity. However, during the times she was not at her best an approach like we used with Clara simply would not have been effective - during those periods she was not attending to environmental cues or feedback and had great difficulty maintaining her attention even on the task itself. Also, even at her best Mary was a person whose competencies were more based in procedural (doing) memory and long established habit patterns and routines than in a more dynamic problem solving based interaction with her environment. Within her own way of doing things she was in many ways more competent than Clara - she was regularly baking things like apple pies for example, but at the same time she was less adaptable and less aware of the activity on a more planned, conscious level, and as such she would not have found it easy to adapt to changes in how she did things - in fact any significant change would tend to throw her off her particular "pathway" through the activity. So it was important for the intervention to enable her to keep her eyes on the path ahead so to speak and not to try and lead her up other routes. We can also construe this within the context of the concept of person-environment. Essentially Mary had developed over many many years a particular relationship with her world that worked for her. But because of the ways dementia had affected her cognition this relationship had become quite rigid - it worked but only under a limited set of conditions. To change those conditions could have changed the whole nature of her relationship with her environment - it would have pushed the world away from her whereas a "just so" intervention based on a full understanding of her range of strengths and limitations enabled the intervention to fit her world better and maintain that connection with it for as long as possible.

Then there was Norma, a lady who had gradually become deskilled over several years of cognitive deterioration that had gone largely unnoticed and entirely unsupported - during which she had, through the repeated experience of not being able to carry out tasks she had once managed independently, developed an overwhelming fear of failure and powerlessness. For Norma cooking was not a valued role - she had become highly restricted in the range of activities she maintained and only used the cooker to heat up hot water (for tea) and soup (which was just about all she ate apart from biscuits). So the intervention (which involved reducing the number of knobs on the cooker to one and ensuring she could only attend to the one corresponding ring) was more about helping her to hold onto the things she was still able to do best for herself, and making them less likely to further provoke her feelings of failure, by reducing the amount of extra demands in the environment and in the task itself (what is referred to as 'environmental press').

Of course I can think of many other situations where the same risk has presented itself and people have been provided with "isolator" switches to temporarily disable the cooker when there is no supervision present, or where others may have had a cooker taken away or replaced with an electric model. In some situations, I have felt it entirely appropriate to have a cooker disabled - but again it's important to reflect on why that may be in some situations, and with some people, but not in others. For example, I can think of people who had long since stopped using the cooker to cook with, but who had begun to explore their environments in a very tactile way and this had led to fiddling with cooker knobs quite inadvertently. In those situations it was clear that it would not be at all disabling to arrange for the cooker to be isolated or taken away completely. This is the crux of the matter: we should ensure that what we do is enabling the person and not contributing further to their deskilling and disablement. In each case we are aiming for an intervention that is at a 'just so' level - i.e. *within* the person's zone of proximal development. The intervention chosen should be one that is not so far removed from their range of abilities and usual way of doing things that it de-skills or disables them further.

For example, getting it wrong might mean making the task too complex or different (e.g. where well meaning carers have bought an electric cooker to replace a gas one, only to find that the person has ended up giving up cooking completely or become even less safe because the cooker is too unfamiliar for them to get used too). Alternatively getting it wrong might mean making it too easy (e.g., as with Clara, we might want the person to continue to attend to environment and task based cues in the process of cooking so as to maintain those vital skills so we would enhance the cues available instead of providing something that does the job for them (such as an automatic sensor/cut-off, which for this reason was felt to be inappropriate for Clara) which would instead remove that stimulus from them and could ultimately contribute to de-skilling them further). So - we need to ensure that such interventions are considered within the context of a high quality, detailed, person-centred assessment process that takes into accounts wishes, approaches, abilities (range of under different conditions) and life history, and we also need, as a result of that process, to be able to make informed judgements about the appropriate level to pitch the intervention at. This is where the concept of Zones of Proximal development becomes most relevant to assessment for assistive technologies (or for that matter any adaptation of task or environment). We are aiming for interventions to provide the person with a 'just so' level of support so as to enable them to carry out their preferred activities and occupations without experiencing a reduction in their sense of agency and mastery or experiencing repeated 'failure' to complete them successfully.

So for Clara, interventions and prompts were kept as minimal as possible and aimed at a level that gave her just enough support to carry out the activity without experiencing a sense of failure, but not so much that she felt we were taking over from her or invalidating her. Just as it is important to maintain a flow of conversation when interacting meaningfully on a social level, so, too, is there a flow process in carrying out an activity. So we always aimed to keep interactions during cooking natural and genuine, making the process a relaxed and realistic one and helping her as much as possible to capitalise on her procedural skills and normal routines,

thus maintaining the flow of the activity and its integrity as a process.

At the end of this assessment/ intervention phase Clara decided that while she wished to prepare her own snacks that she was finding more complex preparation of main meals a chore herself, so was provided with homecare once daily to do that. She was happy with that as she was also getting a lot out of having regular visitors. It was more important to Clara that she have time to herself to use as she chose than to be fully independent in everything, so this was a good balance for her. On the other hand if homecare had been doing all meals for her, as had originally been the recommendation, she would have found this too intrusive as it would have taken away not so much a valued skill and role but more her freedom to live as she wanted and not be tied to other people's schedules. So maintaining some independence cooking snacks was still important.

It's important to understand that when working in this way with someone that assessment is not just about what that person can or cannot do. Scaffolding is a means of assessment and intervention combined as a dialectical process - it is more fundamentally about *what we are doing ourselves* to help support the person in that activity. Reflection on our own approach, such as our language or how we are providing cues, and on what we are contributing to the task, enables a detailed assessment to be made of how we might support the person better. For example, while working with Clara in preparing meals it became apparent that she needed more visual cues to help her notice what she was doing. Some of these could be devolved back to the environment through the provision of written cues and markers on the cooker in order to provide a remnant of our social structure for when we were no longer around. In a way it was about rebuilding a routine and structure with Clara that worked for her; making it another pathway. This was a key part of the grading process; it was about exploring ways for Clara to master certain elements of the task to the best of her abilities, and exploring ways to devolve aspects she still needed support in to the social/physical environment, whether through provision of cues and prompts or an element of social care and continued support. This collaborative reflective process was therefore also a process *of goal setting and negotiation;* discussion not just of what to maintain but what she felt she could let go of. It also facilitated an adjustment process through enabling her to 'reality test' in a supportive environment. For example, at the end of two weeks of assessment in relation to cooking meals, Clara decided that while she wished to prepare her own snacks that she found more involved cooking a chore herself so was provided with homecare to do that. She was happy with that as she was also getting a lot out of having regular visitors. It was more important to Clara that she have time to herself to use as she chose than to be fully independent in everything so this was a good balance for her. On the other hand if homecare had been doing all meals for her she would have found this too intrusive as it would have taken away not so much a valued skill and role (as in Mary's case), but more her freedom to live as she wanted and not be tied to other people's schedules, so maintaining some independence cooking snacks was vitally important to her. Finally the process was also based around a *relationship*, there was a process of getting to know Clara and how she functioned within her environment and her social world, her life history and helping her make best use of the approaches she had developed herself that enabled her to function optimally.

A social-ecological framework for dementia rehabilitation

Clara returned home two years ago and despite having been seen as someone who should probably not go back home in the first place was still managing at home when I last spoke to her family. Revealingly, when followed up some weeks after returning home by the psychiatrist she had only improved in terms of a MMSE score by a couple of points. Initially I was a little surprised by this, as she was now better oriented than previously. However, on the whole this score made sense. Many of the skills Clara was maintaining operated on a very 'procedural' level, they were all to do with 'doing' things, with habit patterns and routines. Not the sort of functional improvements the MMSE is really able to measure sensitively. Creating the right conditions for the person to function optimally often means helping the person make the most of those areas, such as procedural skills, that remain most intact.

Working with people 'in the zone' means assessment and treatment are a dynamic and interactive process with the relationship and partnership established with the person at its centre. The emphasis of assessment and treatment is no longer on the isolated individual, what they can and can't manage 'independently', but on the person within the context of their relationships with their environment, and most importantly, how that relationship is mediated socially - i.e. by ourselves, and by their life history and culture.

Although it is important to identify strengths and needs there is a danger that doing this can strip them from their meaningful context as they are expressed socially and culturally. It is important to recognise that in the real world skills do not exist in a vacuum, they are an expression of Personhood, embedded in social roles, routines, life history, and well being. Working in the person's zone of proximal development means what is often more important is not just to assess strengths and needs (which are of course both *outside* of the Zone) but to identify *points of transition*; emergent processes where opportunities for therapeutic engagement are most likely to be found and where such interventions are most likely to have a meaning and relevance to the person with dementia. This Vygotskian perspective also teaches us that while formal methods of assessment within a rehabilitative context - such as standardised tools - is a useful starting point in determining the individual's current level of independent functioning, this in itself is not necessarily going to be an accurate predictor of their ability to respond to intervention - i.e. their potential. There is arguably a greater need for dynamic assessment tools and approaches, although in my experience much can also be achieved by using standardised tools in new ways. Because Scaffolding is based around shared activity, some of the most useful tools I have found in setting interventions at the correct level are to make use of a detailed process activity analysis and synthesis. This sort of 'dialectical' or dynamic process of assessment enables interventions to engage with the person at the point they will most benefit from them, *within* the Zone of Proximal Development, *not* under or outside of it.

Conclusions - implications for dementia rehab.

As with the "sensitive caregiver" described by Kitwood, we also need to work sensitively and collaboratively with what the person has to offer, to help create conditions that bring out the best they have to offer, and as much as possible help bring the world back within their grasp practically, conceptually and meaningfully. To me this is the essence of dementia rehabilitation. Contrary to those who argue people with dementia are 'not suitable' for rehabilitation I would argue that rehabilitation is possible at every point in the dementia process. In fact I agree strongly with Kitwood's view concerning facilitatory practice, which he referred to as 'positive person work':

> *'The greater the degree of NI (neurological impairment), the more PPW (positive person work) is provided. This is the very opposite of what has traditionally happened'.*

> Kitwood, (1997)

In every person experiencing dementia and at every point along its course there are contradictory processes at work. This is due to a combination of factors. Firstly what Kitwood described as the "dialectics" of dementia. Dementia is not reducible to a process of neurological impairment alone, but is compounded by dynamic interaction with factors such as the individuals own personality and life history, psychological factors such as mood, motivation, anxiety and volition, fluctuations in the person's state of health (or that of their carer's), and the psycho-social environment that they are part of. We should also remember that on a deeper, more fundamental level people are still growing and developing "as people" whatever age and whatever the state of their health. Processes of resolution and integration including what is simplistically described as "new learning" are possible I would argue at any age and any stage of the dementia process. Kitwood described such processes as "Rementia". A therapeutic approach at its heart is about creating and re-creating the conditions that facilitate growth and integration.

Secondly, on a neurological level alone there are also contradictory process at work (interacting dynamically with the other levels already described). As well as whatever processes are contributing to a breakdown of neurological function, whether this be due to formation of plaques and tangles, vascular deterioration or infarcts, there are also processes of neuroplasticity and neuro-integration seeking to repair function and compensate for deficits. This is a dynamic and adaptive process. The question for rehabilitation is how can we tap into and facilitate such processes? Today we also have a number of drugs that can slow down aspects of the dementia process for suitable individuals, at least temporarily, and in the near future we may also have drugs that can facilitate aspects of neuroplasticity and integration. I would argue that rehabilitation can and should play an integral role in memory services helping people to make the best use of whatever benefits such drugs have to offer. Any cognitive benefit arising from taking a drug like Aricept is largely meaningless unless it is incorporated into tangible benefits to the individual in the context of their everyday existence, practical functioning and quality of life. A process of rehabilitation based in a

Scaffolding approach can help identify the best level to engage with the person therapeutically that will facilitate this.

Thirdly, a social-ecological approach places each person within the context of their social relations and culture. Phenomena like memory, cognition, skills and personhood are not the property of isolated individuals but individuals that exist in a lived, historical relationship with others: one that can be enabling and supportive, or that can further contribute to disability and dis-integration. The work that Kitwood carried out helped to expose the many, often subtle, sometimes explicit, ways that society can disable and exclude individuals with dementia. The conceptual framework I have described above based on the work of Vygotsky, shows how we also need to develop an understanding of how social support systems and the psycho-social environment can be enabling, empowering and inclusive and how this can help form the basis of a positive rehabilitative and therapeutic approach to the person with dementia.

References and further reading

Cole, M., 1985 *The Zone of Proximal Development: Where Culture and Cognition Create Each Other.* in Wertsch, J., (1985) Culture, Communication and Cognition. Cambridge: Cambridge University Press.

Greenberg Lyons, B., (1984) *Defining a Child's Zone of Proximal Development: Evaluation Process for Treatment Planning.* American Journal of Occupational Therapy. 38/7, p.446-451

Lawton, M.P., & Nahemow, L.E., (1973) *Ecology and the Ageing process.* In Eisdorfer, C., & Lawton,

M.P., (eds.), The Psychology of Adult Development and Ageing (pp 619-674). Washington DC: American Psychological Association

Kitwood, T., (1990) *Psychotherapy and Dementia.* Psychotherapy Section Newsletter. 8. p40-56

Kitwood, T., (1993) *Towards a Theory of Dementia Care: The Interpersonal Process.* Ageing and Society. 13, p51-67.

Kitwood, T., (1997) Dementia Reconsidered: The person comes first. Buckingham: Open University Press.

Luria, A.R., (1979) The Making of Mind. Harvard University Press.

Meadows, S., (1993) The Child as a Thinker: The development and acquisition of cognition in childhood. London, Routledge.

Meadows, S., (1996) Parenting Behaviour and Children's Cognitive Development. Psychology Press.

Saloman, G., (ed). (1993) Distributed Cognitions: Psychological and Educational Implications. Cambridge: Cambridge University Press.

Seely Brown, J, Collins, A., & Duguid, P., *(1989) Situated Cognition and the Culture of Learning.* Educational Researcher; v.18 no.1, pp. 32-42.

Wertsch, J.V., (1985) Vygotsky and the Social Formation of Mind. Harvard University Press.

Wertsch, J.V., (1998) Mind as Action. Oxford: Oxford University Press.

Wey, S., (2002) *Intensive Home Based Dementia Rehabilitation.* Journal of Dementia Care. 10 (3) 28-33

Wey, S., (2004) *One Size Does Not Fit All.* In Perspectives on Rehabilitation and Dementia. Marshall, M., (ed). London, Jessica Kingsley.

Vygotsky, L.S., (1978) Mind in Society: The Development of Higher Psychological Processes. Harvard University Press.

A note on contributors

John Woolham works as a Senior Research Officer for Northamptonshire County Council. Shortly after gaining a D.Phil from Sussex University he worked at a Community Mental Health Centre in Sussex before working in Northamptonshire. He was a member of the ASTRID project team and contributed to the ASTRID Guide. After this he was jointly responsible for setting up the Safe at Home project in Northamptonshire - the first project in England and Wales to use technology to support people with dementia and their carers. He has published a number of studies in this field. He is currently a member of the National Telecare Advisory Group for England.
Contact:
jwoolham@northamptonshire.gov.uk

Marilyn Cash has worked with older people and people with dementia in both the voluntary and statutory sectors, in social care and as a researcher. Her research on assistive technology was undertaken whilst she was working with Dementia Voice, Bristol (the Dementia Services. Development Centre for South-West England). She is particularly interested in allowing the 'voice' of older people including those with dementia to be heard in research and for research to be made accessible to those groups.
Contact:
m_cash2@yahoo.co.uk.

Christine Calder works as a Resource Worker for South Lanarkshire Council where she is a member of the Older Peoples Services Headquarters Team. She has spent a number of years working with older people in elderly forums and campaigning groups before moving on to working within the field of community care. She has lead responsibility for the development of assistive technology within older people's services in South Lanarkshire She is a member of the Technology Interest Group which is led by the Dementia Services Centre at Stirling University.
Contact:
Christine.calder@southlanarkshire.gov.uk

Dyllis Faife has interests and expertise in the areas of stroke, dementia care, assistive technology and joint working between health and social services. She continues to play a leading role in the development, organisation and management of electronic assistive technology in Norfolk Social Services. She established, and currently chairs, 'Dementia Focus' – a regional centre of expertise in dementia care across Norfolk, Suffolk and Cambridgeshire. She was a member of the Department of Health Policy Collaborative for Electronic technology and is a member of the National Care Workforce Group for Older People.
Contact:
Dyllis.faife@norfolk.gov.uk

Eileen Askham is Director of Care Services with FOLD Housing Association in Northern Ireland and acts as Consultant to the newly formed Fold Ireland Housing Association in the Republic of Ireland. Appointed to her present post in 1993, she has full responsibility for the management of FOLD's Special Needs Housing and Care Schemes, Day Care Services, the 'Staying Put' Home Improvement Service, and Fold's TeleCare service.
She is a member of the Registration and Conduct Committee of the new Northern Ireland Social Care Council and a Board member of The Link Family and Community Centre.
Contact:
Eileen.askham@foldgroup.co.uk

Clive Baldwin is Senior Lecturer in Dementia Studies and Course Co-ordinator for the MSc distance learning programme. He trained as a social worker in 1991 and worked in a variety of community development posts in the voluntary sector. He completed his PhD in Sociology in 2000 with research focused on Munchausen syndrome by proxy. His research and academic interests are ethics and dementia, narrative theory and method and dementia and technology. He is also a member of the Christian Council on Ageing Dementia Group.
Contact:
P.C.Baldwin@bradford.ac.uk

Michael Mandelstam previously worked in the voluntary sector and then at the Department of Health. Now working independently he provides legal training, consultancy and advice to local authorities and the NHS. He is a author of a number of books on aspects of community care law, including Community Care Practice and the Law (3rd edition, 2005).
Contact:
michael.mandelstam@btinternet.com.

Steven Wey works as a Senior occupational therapist for Leeds Community Mental Health Trust. At the present time he works on an acute assessment/treatment ward for people with dementia. Before this, he worked in a pioneering home assessment, treatment and rehabilitation team for people with dementia. Prior to becoming an Occupational Therapist in 1993 he worked at different times in nursing, journalism and the voluntary sector.
Contact:
Stephen.wey@leedsmh.nhs.uk